work manual for introductory **maternity nursing**

FIFTH EDITION

Doris C. Bethea
R.N., B.S., M.S.

Formerly Clinical Specialist, Maternity Nursing, and Instructor,
Practical Nursing Program, Porter Memorial Hospital,
Denver, Colorado; Assistant Professor of Nursing,
Union College, Lincoln, Nebraska

J. B. LIPPINCOTT COMPANY
Philadelphia
London • Mexico City • New York • St. Louis • São Paulo • Sydney

Sponsoring Editor: Nancy Mullins
Manuscript Editor: Linda J. Stewart
Design Coordinator: Anita Curry
Designer: Adrianne Onderdonk Dudden
Cover Design: Kevin Curry
Production Manager: Kathleen P. Dunn
Compositor: McFarland Graphics
Printer/Binder: Malloy Lithographing
Cover Printer: Lehigh Press

5th Edition

6 5 4

Any procedure or practice described in this book should be applied by the health-care practitioner under appropriate supervision in accordance with professional standards of care used with regard to the unique circumstances that apply in each practice situation. Care has been taken to confirm the accuracy of information presented and to describe generally accepted practices. However, the author, editors and publisher cannot accept any responsibility for errors or omissions or for consequences from application of the information in this book and make no warranty, express or implied, with respect to the contents of the book.

Every effort has been made to ensure drug selections and dosages are in accordance with current recommendations and practice. Because of ongoing research, changes in government regulations and the constant flow of information on drug therapy, reactions and interactions, the reader is cautioned to check the package insert for each drug for indications, dosages, warnings and precautions, particularly if the drug is new or infrequently used.

preface

This workbook has been prepared to accompany the fifth edition of *Introductory Maternity Nursing*. The major portion of the workbook consists of simulated patient situations with multiple choice questions; it also contains occasional matching sets in basic vocabulary and concepts. Answers to the questions are included to aid the student in self-evaluation.

It is anticipated that the workbook will help to reinforce the student's knowledge of important facts and help her transfer her basic knowledge to clinical situations. The multiple choice questions afford extra practice for State Board examinations.

Doris C. Bethea, R.N., B.S., M.S.

contents

the family in modern 1 society

I. **SITUATION:** Jason is a 10-year-old boy adopted by a married couple who lives on a farm. They have two other adopted children, a 12-year-old boy and a 6-year-old girl.

Place the letter of the *best* answer in the space before the statement.

__D__
1. You would expect that Jason would receive from his new family
   (1) love
   (2) discipline
   (3) moral values
   (4) life skills
   (5) security
   A. (1) and (5)
   B. All except (4)
   C. All except (3)
   D. All of these

__B__
2. The type of family to which Jason now belongs is
   A. a social contract family
   B. a nuclear family
   C. a single parent family
   D. an extended family

__C__
3. Which of the benefits usually provided by belonging to a family is Jason *least* likely to receive from adoption into this family?
   A. love
   B. discipline
   C. pride in his ancestry
   D. security

__C__
4. The importance of the family to the individual and to society cannot be stressed too much. Which of the following effects does the family have on society?
   (1) provides stability
   (2) sets standards and values
   (3) provides guidelines for social interaction
   (4) promotes cultural growth
   (5) promotes responsible behavior
   A. (2) and (4) only
   B. (1), (3), and (5)
   C. All of these
   D. None of these

A variety of life-styles have recently evolved as individuals have rejected traditional values and have sought to establish life-styles based on their own values and desires. Which of the following would be considered evolving life-styles?

__D__
5. **(1)** traditional family
   (2) social contract family
   (3) commune family
   (4) single parent family
   (5) extended family
   A. All of these
   B. (1), (2), and (5)
   C. (3), (4), and (5)
   D. (2), (3), and (4)

_B_ **6.** Health workers providing care to individuals with nontraditional lifestyles are more likely to be effective if they realize that these individuals
   (1) are usually well educated
   (2) require fuller and more complete explanations than other patients
   (3) may reject advice
   (4) are usually from the lower socioeconomic group
   (5) will accept without question advice and information
   A. (1) only
   B. (1), (2), and (3)
   C. (4) only
   D. (2), (4), and (5)

_C_ **7.** A family consisting of a legally married husband and wife and their children is called
   A. an extended family
   B. a social contract family
   C. a nuclear family
   D. a commune family

_B_ **8.** A family consisting of a man and woman living together without legal sanctions is
   A. an extended family
   B. a social contract family
   C. a nuclear family
   D. a single parent family

_A_ **9.** Single parents may spend so much of their time parenting and earning a living for themselves and their children that they may
   A. disregard their own social and personal growth needs
   B. disregard their children's needs for their attention
   C. lose interest in their jobs
   D. develop stronger coping abilities

ANSWERS · CHAPTER 1

I. **1.** D   **4.** C   **7.** C
   2. B   **5.** D   **8.** B
   3. C   **6.** B   **9.** A

the family and 2 pregnancy

I. SITUATION: Debbie is a 28-year-old woman who has completed college and is employed at a bank. Her 30-year-old husband, Bob, is also a college graduate with a job as an electronics engineer. They have been married for 5 years and are expecting their first baby. They delayed beginning their family until they were able to make a substantial down payment on a new home in the suburbs. This pregnancy was planned and is definitely desired. Their insurance will cover the usual expenses of pregnancy.

Place the letter of the *best* answer in the space before the statement.

_D_ 1. When Debbie first suspected that she was pregnant, she probably
    A. tried to postpone awareness of it
    B. attempted to deny it
    C. thought she had the "flu"
    D. thought it was too good to be true

_A_ 2. Bob went with Debbie on her first visit to the obstetrician. When the doctor told him that "it looks like you're going to be a daddy," you would expect Bob's response to be one of
    A. happiness
    B. disappointment
    C. acceptance
    D. resignation

_D_ 3. Since this is their first pregnancy, Debbie and Bob do not have to consider attitudes of other children toward the pregnancy. If they did, they could promote positive attitudes by
    (1) being pleased with the pregnancy
    (2) explaining to the children early how the expected child will fit into the family
    (3) including them in the planning for the new baby
    (4) making necessary changes in the home to accommodate the new baby gradually
    A. All except (1)
    B. All except (4)
    C. (2) and (3)
    D. All of these

_B_ 4. Although Debbie's entire life will be affected to some extent by her pregnancy, which will probably be most obvious?
    A. diet and clothing
    B. appearance and feelings
    C. sexual responses and desires
    D. job, social, and recreational activities

_C_ 5. Which of the following will probably cause Debbie the *least* concern during this pregnancy?
    A. her appearance
    B. mood swings
    C. finances
    D. normal discomforts of pregnancy

_D_ **6.** In addition to the longed-for child, another desirable outcome Debbie may receive from pregnancy is
  A. a deeper and more meaningful relationship with her husband
  B. increased emotional growth and maturity
  C. an increased capacity for caring for others
  D. all of these

_B_ **7.** Probably the best way Bob can grow and mature emotionally during this pregnancy is by providing Debbie with
  A. economic security
  B. emotional support and companionship
  C. physical needs and comforts
  D. social and recreational activities

_A_ **8.** In your contacts with Bob, you may be able to help by explaining beforehand the types of feelings he may experience during the pregnancy. In addition to his feelings of happiness, there may be times when he will feel
  (1) jealous
  (2) unable to cope
  (3) insecure
  (4) bewildered
  A. All of these
  B. All except (1)
  C. All except (2)
  D. (3) and (4)

_B_ **9.** The effect pregnancy has on children in the family depends to a great extent on their
  A. size
  B. age
  C. sex
  D. activities

_B_ **10.** Probably the least desirable effect the children will experience from the pregnancy will be due to the mother's
  A. trips to the doctor
  B. mood changes
  C. morning sickness
  D. desires concerning the sex of the new baby

_C_ **11.** Debbie's decision to breast-feed the baby depends upon
  (1) her own personal feelings and preferences
  (2) Bob's feelings and wishes
  (3) her doctor's advice
  (4) whether or not she plans to continue working
  A. (1) only
  B. (1) and (4)
  C. All of these
  D. (2) and (3)

_A_ **12.** Parents who decide to formula-feed the infant should know that
  (1) inexpensive formula can be prepared using evaporated milk, Karo, and water
  (2) it is important to the baby's emotional well-being that he be held while fed
  (3) the infant's nutritional needs can be met satisfactorily with formula
  (4) prepared formula is available
  A. All of these
  B. (2) only
  C. (1) and (3)
  D. All except (4)

_D_ **13.** The teenage father may need counseling regarding
  (1) preparation for fatherhood
  (2) contraception
  (3) responsible sexuality
  (4) job training
  (5) caretaking decisions
  A. (1) and (3)
  B. (1) and (4)
  C. All except (2)
  D. All of these

<u>B</u> **14.** The psychological tasks the pregnant woman accomplishes during pregnancy are progressive steps in her emotional adjustment to the pregnancy. One task is usually completed in each trimester of pregnancy. During the first trimester the task is
  A. acceptance of the fetus as a being separate from herself
  B. acceptance of the pregnancy
  C. to get ready for the birth
  D. to realize that she is going to be a parent

<u>A</u> **15.** The task accomplished during the second trimester is
  A. acceptance of the fetus as a being separate from herself
  B. acceptance of the pregnancy
  C. to get ready for the birth
  D. to realize that she is going to be a parent

II. In the space before the description of clothing for the infant in Column I, place the letter of the quality that it fits in Column II.

I	II
DESCRIPTION OF INFANT'S CLOTHING	QUALITY

<u>A</u> **1.** Soft   **A.** Comfortable

<u>B</u> **2.** Material that can take repeated washings   **B.** Practical

<u>B</u> **3.** Good material

<u>A</u> **4.** Smooth seams

<u>A</u> **5.** Warm for winter, cool for summer

<u>B</u> **6.** Adequate size so as not to be outgrown too soon

<u>A</u> **7.** No frills around the neck

<u>A</u> **8.** Not constricting

<u>B</u> **9.** Made well

III. In Column I list the items Debbie should take to the hospital for her personal use. In Column II list the items Debbie should take for bringing the baby home.

I	II
Toiletries	Undershirt
Bras	Diapers
Gown	Outfit to come home in
Robe & slippers	Blankets
Clothes to wear home	Booties, Bonnet or cap

IV. Since this is Debbie and Bob's first pregnancy, list at least two potential nursing diagnoses that might be appropriate for them.
  1.

  2.

I. 1. D   5. C   9. B   13. D
    2. A   6. D   10. B   14. B
    3. D   7. B   11. C   15. A
    4. B   8. A   12. A

II. 1. A   4. A   7. A
    2. B   5. A   8. A
    3. B   6. B   9. B

III. See Chapter 2 of *Introductory Maternity Nursing,* 5th edition.

IV. 1. Knowledge deficit related to pregnancy and how it can affect one's feelings
    2. Anxiety related to fulfilling their role as parents
    3. Disturbance in self-concept and body-image related to changes in Debbie's appearance

the past and present in 3 maternity care

I. Place the letter of the *best* answer in the space before the statement.

___C___   **1.** The first cesarean section on a live patient was performed in 1610 by
   A. Palfyne
   B. Johan Peter Frank
   C. Trautmann of Wittenberg
   D. Raynaldes

___A___   **2.** Official credit for the invention of obstetric forceps in 1770 is given to
   A. Palfyne
   B. Johan Peter Frank
   C. Raynaldes
   D. Peter Chamberlen

___D___   **3.** It is known that obstetric forceps were used prior to the 16th century by the
   A. Hebrews
   B. Greeks
   C. Romans
   D. Egyptians

___B___   **4.** It is believed that obstetric forceps were invented in 1580 and kept as a family secret by
   A. Palfyne
   B. Peter Chamberlen
   C. Roesslin
   D. William Smellie

___A___   **5.** In the 18th century, forceps were improved by the addition of a steel lock and curved blades. These changes were made by
   A. William Smellie
   B. Louis Pasteur
   C. Hendrik Van Deventer
   D. Oliver Wendell Holmes

___C___   **6.** The first English textbook on obstetrics was
   A. *The Cause, Concept and Prophylaxis of Puerperal Fever* by Semmelweis
   B. *Lex Regis* by Julius Caesar
   C. *Byrthe of Mankynd* by Raynaldes
   D. *Ta Sheng P'Ien* by Lee Hwang

___A___   **7.** The first person in this country to accurately describe the nature of puerperal sepsis and to establish guidelines to prevent the disease was
   A. Oliver Wendell Holmes
   B. Ignaz Philipp Semmelweis
   C. Hendrik Van Deventer
   D. Sir James Y. Simpson

_D_ **8.** The German who believed that all childbirth should be attended by trained persons and that state aid should be provided to the newly delivered mother so that she could have time to recuperate and care for her baby, and spread his belief through his writings between 1779 and 1817, was
   A. Roesslin
   B. William Smellie
   C. Raynaldes
   D. Johan Peter Frank

_B_ **9.** The man who is called the father of modern obstetrics is
   A. William Smellie
   B. Hendrik Van Deventer
   C. Ignaz Philipp Semmelweis
   D. Oliver Wendell Holmes

_C_ **10.** The man, in Vienna, who proved the nature of the source and transmission of puerperal sepsis was
   A. Sir James Y. Simpson
   B. Louis Pasteur
   C. Ignaz Phillipp Semmelweis
   D. Kalletschka

_A_ **11.** In 1879, doctors were first shown the organism which caused puerperal fever, and aseptic technique was recommended as the way to control its spread by
   A. Louis Pasteur
   B. Kalletschka
   C. Oliver Wendell Holmes
   D. William Smellie

_D_ **12.** The first anesthetic used in obstetrics was in 1847 by
   A. Oliver Wendell Holmes
   B. Ignaz Philipp Semmelweis
   C. Hendrik Van Deventer
   D. Sir James Y. Simpson

_C_ **13.** The first anesthetic used in obstetrics was
   A. chloroform
   B. nitrous oxide
   C. ether
   D. pentothal

_B_ **14.** Queen Victoria's contribution to obstetrics consisted of silencing some of the opponents of anesthesia for obstetrics when she
   A. accepted ether for delivery in 1853
   B. accepted chloroform for delivery in 1853
   C. published an article favoring anesthesia for obstetrics in 1853
   D. jailed the opponents of anesthesia for obstetrics in 1853

_D_ **15.** Recent developments in obstetrics include
   (1) technology to diagnose and treat fetal conditions in utero
   (2) in vitro fertilization and embryo transplants
   (3) technology that saves the lives of all preterm infants that weigh at least 600 to 700 g
   (4) measures to prevent the birth of preterm infants
   (5) choices in the type of facilities and services available to expectant couples
   A. All of these
   B. All except (4)
   C. (2), (3), and (4)
   D. (1), (2), and (5)

_B_ **16.** A new type of maternity care facility that provides a home-like atmosphere for childbirth and permits the mother to labor, give birth, recover, and spend her postpartum hospital stay in the same room is
   A. a birthing room
   B. a single unit facility
   C. the traditional facility
   D. an ABC

_____ **17.** Alternative birthing centers

   (1) permit choice of place of birth, plan of care, and persons present at birth
   (2) provide a homelike atmosphere
   (3) provide medical safety
   (4) are restricted to low-risk women
   (5) require participants to attend expectant parents' classes
   A. (1) only
   B. All except (3)
   C. (1), (2), and (5)
   D. All of these

II. PROJECTS

   1. Find out what facilities are available to expectant couples in your area: the traditional hospital setting, birthing rooms, ABCs, single unit facilities?
   2. How soon are preterm infants discharged from hospitals in your area?
   3. What is the average length of stay for maternity patients in your area?
   4. Is there follow-up care (telephone? home visits?) by hospital nurses for parents of preterm infants and/or postpartum patients who are discharged early?

ANSWERS · CHAPTER 3

I.
1. C
2. A
3. D
4. B
5. A

6. C
7. A
8. D
9. B
10. C

11. A
12. D
13. C
14. B
15. D

16. B
17. D

the nursing process in **4** maternity care

I. Explain the difference between:

A. Obstetrics and maternity nursing _____
_____
_____

B. Family practice physicians and obstetricians _____
_____
_____

C. Family practice physicians and pediatricians _____
_____
_____

D. Obstetricians and residents _____
_____
_____

E. Midwives and nurse-midwives _____
_____
_____

F. Neonatal death and fetal death _____
_____
_____

II. Before the term in Column I, place the letter of the item in Column II that best describes it.

I

_H_ **1.** Birth rate
_F_ **2.** Marriage rate
_D_ **3.** Fertility rate
_A_ **4.** Neonatal death rate
_C_ **5.** Infant mortality rate
_G_ **6.** Perinatal mortality rate
_E_ **7.** Maternal mortality rate

II

A. Number of infant deaths during the first 4 weeks after birth per 1,000 births

B. Number of maternal deaths per 1,000 live births

C. Number of infant deaths before the first birthday per 1,000 live births

D. Number of births per 1,000 women between 15 and 44 years of age

E. Number of maternal deaths per 100,000 live births

F. Number of marriages per 1,000 population

G. Number of deaths of fetuses and infants weighing 1,000 g or more which occur between 28 weeks' gestation and 4 weeks of age

H. Number of births per 1,000 population

III. Complete the sentence by filling the blank with the correct term from the list below.

General hospitals
Homes for retarded children
Children's hospitals
Genetic counseling centers
Hyde Amendment
Public health departments
Adoption agencies
Planned Parenthood Association
National Office of Vital Statistics
U.S. Children's Bureau

1. _Children's hospitals_ are especially equipped to care for premature infants and other infants born with acute problems.

2. _Adoption agencies_ are important both to the unwed mother who wishes to relinquish her baby and to the couple who wishes to adopt a child.

3. _U S C B_ was established in 1912 during the administration of President Theodore Roosevelt.

4. _P P A_ offers services and information to couples who wish to limit the size of their families and to space their pregnancies.

5. Functions of _Public health Dept_ include setting standards for care, case finding, follow-up care on referrals, conducting antepartal and postpartal clinics, well-baby clinics, and family planning clinics.

6. _N O V S_ compiles studies dealing with the birth rate, marriage rate, infant mortality rate etc.

7. The _Hyde amendment_ limits use of federal funds for abortion.

IV. SITUATION: Debbie and Bob are both employed in responsible positions and they both enjoy their jobs. They delayed beginning their family until they were able to make a good down payment on their new home and to put aside some money in a savings account.

Place the letter of the *best* answer in the space before the statement.

_A_ **1.** You would expect that the maternity care Debbie receives would be provided by
  A. an obstetrician
  B. a pediatrician
  C. a resident
  D. a midwife

_E_ **2.** If the aim of maternity care is to be realized for this couple,
- **(1)** Debbie must go through pregnancy, labor, and birth with minimal discomfort and optimal health
- **(2)** their expected child must receive optimal care
- **(3)** they must develop wholesome attitudes toward family relationships
- **(4)** they must be aware of the responsibilities of parenthood
- **(5)** they must develop judgment and abilities to meet the responsibilities of parenthood in a confident and satisfying manner
- **A.** (1) only
- **B.** (2) only
- **C.** (4) and (5)
- **D.** All except (3)
- **E.** All of these

_D_ **3.** Age is one of the factors that influences the number of women who become recipients of maternity care. Most births occur among women who are between the ages of
- **A.** 15 and 19
- **B.** 20 and 24
- **C.** 25 and 29
- **D.** 20 and 29

_B_ **4.** The safest time for women to give birth appears to be between the ages of
- **A.** 15 and 19
- **B.** 20 and 24
- **C.** 25 and 29
- **D.** 20 and 29

_D_ **5.** Which of the following have resulted from the availability of acceptable methods of birth control?
- **(1)** couples are able to postpone beginning their families
- **(2)** couples are able to limit the size of their families
- **(3)** couples are able to space their children
- **(4)** children are being conceived solely as a result of the sexual drive
- **A.** All of these
- **B.** (1), (3), and (4)
- **C.** (2), (3), and (4)
- **D.** (1), (2), and (3)
- **E.** (4) only

_A_ **6.** Legally, a birth certificate must be completed on every birth in
- **A.** all 50 states and the District of Columbia
- **B.** about one half of the states
- **C.** all states except Alaska and Hawaii
- **D.** none of the states

_D_ **7.** The birth certificate is legal proof of
- **(1)** age
- **(2)** citizenship
- **(3)** family relationships
- **(4)** religion
- **A.** All of these
- **B.** (1), (2), and (4)
- **C.** (1), (3), and (4)
- **D.** (1), (2), and (3)

_B_ **8.** The leading causes of maternal mortality in this country are
- **(1)** hemorrhage
- **(2)** pneumonia
- **(3)** infection
- **(4)** pregnancy-induced hypertension
- **A.** (1), (2), and (3)
- **B.** (1), (3), and (4)
- **C.** (2), (3), and (4)
- **D.** All of these

_D_ 9. Some of the advances in maternity care in recent years that have made childbirth safer include
(1) better prepared personnel
(2) better equipped facilities
(3) methods of preventing and treating hemorrhage
(4) methods of preventing and treating infection
(5) better antepartal care
A. (1), (3), and (4)
B. (3), (4), and (5)
C. (2), (3), and (4)
D. All of these
E. All except (5)

_C_ 10. The agency to which all births in this country are reported is the
A. U.S. Children's Bureau
B. public health department
C. National Office of Vital Statistics
D. federal government

_C_ 11. Among the factors which influence the number of women who become pregnant, and therefore recipients of maternity care, are the
(1) marriage rate
(2) number of women in their twenties
(3) desire of a woman to bear a child
(4) availability of acceptable birth control methods
(5) illegitimacy rate
A. All of these
B. All except (3)
C. All except (5)
D. All except (2)

_D_ 12. The nurse can learn about the patient's culture by
(1) asking the patient
(2) visiting in the patient's home
(3) reading about it
(4) listening to the patient
(5) learning the patient's language
A. All of these
B. All except (2)
C. All except (3)
D. All except (5)

_C_ 13. The most important reasons the nurse needs to understand the patient's culture are
(1) so that the nurse can adapt her care to make it more acceptable to the patient
(2) so that the patient will understand the nurse's language
(3) so that the nurse will understand why the patient responds the way she does
(4) so that the nurse can understand the patient's language
(5) because culture affects one's attitudes toward childbearing
A. (1), (2), and (5)
B. (2), (3), and (4)
C. (1), (3), and (5)
D. (3), (4), and (5)

_B_ 14. Which of the following is *not* a step in the nursing process?
A. assessment
B. flow sheet
C. analysis
D. implementation

V. In the space before the definition in Column I, place the letter of the term from Column II that it defines.

	I DEFINITION		II TERM
C	**1.** Involves defining desired or expected goals or outcomes of care, setting priorities, and choosing appropriate actions	**A.**	Assessment
A	**2.** Collection of subjective and objective data regarding the patient and her health problem	**B.**	Analysis
K	**3.** A short form for recording pertinent information; not a legal record; usually discarded after patient is discharged	**C.** **D.**	Planning Implementation
E	**4.** Involves determining the progress made toward reaching desired goals	**E.** **F.**	Evaluation Nursing diagnosis
H	**5.** Records by the nurse of nursing information	**G.**	Data base
M	**6.** Legal guidelines for the nurse in performance of her duties	**H.** **I.**	Nurse's notes Graphic
B	**7.** Interpretation of data; involves judgment and decision-making	**J.** **K.**	Discharge summary Kardex
I	**8.** Short form on which vital signs are graphed	**L.**	Flow sheet
F	**9.** Statement of the patient's problem, treatable by the nurse	**M.** **N.**	Standards of Care Nursing process
L	**10.** A short form used for frequent recordings of vital signs and other aspects of a patient's condition; shows fluctuations and changes at a glance		
D	**11.** Actions or interventions by the nurse to attain desired goals or outcomes		
N	**12.** A way of identifying and solving patient health problems within the scope of nursing practice.		
G	**13.** Contains information obtained when the patient is admitted or first seen; initial assessment by the nurse		
J	**14.** Contains instructions given to the patient and details of follow-up care		

VI. PROJECTS: Using the telephone directory, community resources directory, or other available sources of information, find out:

1. What facilities or agencies for assisting unmarried mothers are available in your community (homes for unmarried mothers, adoption agencies etc.) and who sponsors them

2. What facilities are available for providing medical and hospital care to expectant mothers in underprivileged groups

3. Whether there are genetic counseling centers in your area

4. Where the nearest special facilities for special problems are located, such as regional centers for premature infants and homes for retarded children

5. The address of the local registrar and the fee for obtaining a certified copy of a birth certificate

6. Whether there are educational facilities for preparing nurse-midwives in your city and whether your state gives them legal status to function as nurse-midwives

7. Where the nearest public health department is located, whether it operates antepartal, postpartal, well-baby, and family planning clinics, and how referrals are made to it

8. Whether there is a homemaker service available in your community and its cost

9. Whether there are marriage counseling services in your community

10. Who staffs the offices of the doctors (both family practice physicians and obstetricians) who care for expectant mothers (RNs, LPNs, LVNs etc.)

11. Whether in your community you can obtain pamphlets on maternal and infant care published by the Children's Bureau of HEW

12. Whether there is a Planned Parenthood Association in your community and what services it provides

I. **A.** Obstetrics is medical care of women during pregnancy and labor and for approximately 6 weeks following delivery, while maternity nursing is care provided by the nurse during the same period. Maternity nursing also includes care of the newborn infant.

B. Family practice physicians care for all members of a family; obstetricians care for women during pregnancy and birth and the period immediately following.

C. Family practice physicians provide care for all members of a family, while pediatricians provide care for newborn infants and children.

D. Obstetricians are specialists in maternity care; residents are physicians who are becoming specialists.

E. A midwife may be an untrained person who provides support and care during birth when medical assistance is not available. A nurse-midwife is a professional nurse who has received special education and preparation in midwifery.

F. Neonatal death is death of the infant within the first 4 weeks after birth; fetal death is death in utero after 20 weeks' gestation.

II. **1.** H **4.** A **7.** E
    2. F **5.** C
    3. D **6.** G

III. **1.** Children's hospitals **5.** Public health departments
    2. Adoption agencies **6.** National Office of Vital Statistics
    3. U.S. Children's Bureau **7.** Hyde Amendment
    4. Planned Parenthood Association

IV. **1.** A **5.** D **9.** D **13.** C
    2. E **6.** A **10.** C **14.** B
    3. D **7.** D **11.** C
    4. B **8.** B **12.** D

V. **1.** C **5.** H **9.** F **13.** G
    2. A **6.** M **10.** L **14.** J
    3. K **7.** B **11.** D
    4. E **8.** I **12.** N

the reproductive 5 system

I. From the list below select the correct label for each of the external female reproductive organs in the diagram.

Anus	Labium major	Mons pubis	Urethra
Clitoris	Labium minor	Perineum	Vagina

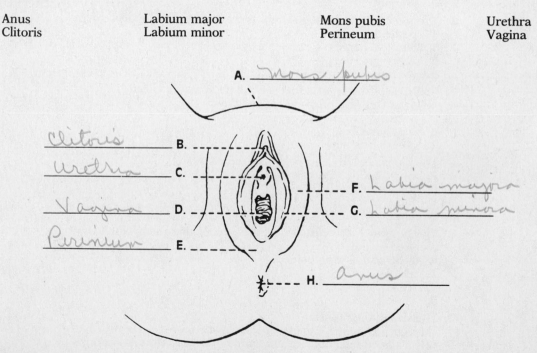

A. _Mons pubis_

Clitoris   B.

Urethra   C.

                F. _Labia majora_

Vagina   D.

                G. _Labia minora_

Perineum   E.

H. _anus_

II. Place the letter of the *best* answer in the space before the statement.

_____ **1.** The female reproductive organ which is comparable to the penis in the male is
    A. vulva
    B. clitoris
    C. hymen
    D. perineum

_D_ 2. Bartholin's glands
   (1) provide a lubricant during sexual activity
   (2) are situated one on either side of the vagina
   (3) are situated one on either side of the urethra
   (4) support the pelvic organs
   A. (1) and (3)
   B. (2) and (4)
   C. (3) and (4)
   D. (1) and (2)

_C_ 3. Collectively, the external female reproductive organs are called the
   A. perineum
   B. vestibule
   C. vulva
   D. mons pubis

_A_ 4. The area extending from the lower border of the vaginal opening downward to the anus is called the
   A. perineum
   B. vestibule
   C. vulva
   D. mons pubis

_C_ 5. The levator ani muscles and fascia, the deep transverse perineal muscles and fascia, and the muscles of the external genitalia
   (1) are enclosed in the vestibule
   (2) make up the perineum
   (3) when intact are evidence of virginity
   (4) provide support for pelvic organs
   A. (1) and (3)
   B. (1) only
   C. (2) and (4)
   D. (3) only

_A_ 6. The muscles, fascia, and skin of the perineum are supplied by the
   A. pudendal nerves
   B. perineal nerves
   C. uterine nerves
   D. ovarian nerves

_D_ 7. The cells of the breasts that secrete the milk are called
   A. tubercles of Montgomery
   B. areola
   C. lobes or lobules
   D. alveoli or acini

_B_ 8. The pigmented area surrounding the nipples is called
   A. tubercles of Montgomery
   B. areola
   C. lobes or lobules
   D. alveoli or acini

_A_ 9. The oil that lubricates the nipples, protecting them when the baby suckles, is secreted by the
   A. tubercles of Montgomery
   B. areola
   C. lobes or lobules
   D. alveoli or acini

_C_ 10. The size of the breasts
   (1) depends on the amount of fatty tissue present
   (2) is a good indication of the amount of milk they will produce
   (3) depends upon the amount of muscle tissue present
   (4) is no indication of the amount of milk they will produce
   A. (1) and (2)
   B. (3) and (4)
   C. (1) and (4)
   D. (2) and (3)

_B_ **11.** During childbirth, the vagina must stretch tremendously to permit passage of the baby. This stretching is possible because the vagina contains
   A. cilia
   B. rugae
   C. muscle
   D. fimbriae

_B_ **12.** Which of the following is *not* a function of the vagina?
   A. it receives the penis during intercourse
   B. it houses the fetus during pregnancy
   C. it is the passageway for menstrual discharges
   D. it is part of the birth canal during delivery

_A_ **13.** In a nonpregnant woman, the size of the uterus is approximately
   A. 1 inch thick × 2 inches wide × 3 inches long
   B. 2 inches thick × 3 inches wide × 4 inches long
   C. 1 inch thick × 3 inches wide × 2 inches long
   D. 2 inches thick × 4 inches wide × 3 inches long

_B_ **14.** The uterus is held in place by ligaments which
   A. keep it from moving
   B. permit its upper portion to move freely
   C. permit its lower portion to move freely
   D. have nothing to do with its ability to move

_D_ **15.** Backache during pregnancy may be caused by the
   A. excessive movement of the baby
   B. excessive size of the baby
   C. pulling and stretching of the cervix
   D. pulling and stretching of the ligaments

_C_ **16.** There are three parts of the uterus. The upper triangular part is called the
   A. cervix
   B. fornix
   C. corpus
   D. fundus

_A_ **17.** The lower cylindrical part of the uterus is called the
   A. cervix
   B. fornix
   C. corpus
   D. fundus

_D_ **18.** The part of the uterus between the fallopian tubes is called the
   A. cervix
   B. fornix
   C. endometrium
   D. fundus

_C_ **19.** The abundant blood supply of the uterus is provided by the
   A. inferior vena cava
   B. ovarian and uterine veins
   C. uterine and ovarian arteries
   D. superior vena cava

_C_ **20.** The muscle fibers of the uterus are arranged to run
   A. in circles
   B. in straight lines
   C. in all directions
   D. parallel to the blood vessels

_A_ **21.** The blood vessels within the uterus are
   A. interwoven among the muscle fibers
   B. parallel to the muscle fibers
   C. located in the endometrium
   D. protected by the mons pubis

_A_ **22.** The purpose of the location of the uterine blood vessels in relation to the muscle fibers is to aid in
   A. controlling hemorrhage following childbirth
   B. supplying adequate oxygen to the fetus
   C. making labor short and painless
   D. making menstruation brief and painless

_D_ **23.** The lining of the uterine cavity is the
  A. perineum
  B. perimetrium
  C. myometrium
  D. endometrium

_A_ **24.** Which of the following is *not* one of the layers of the uterus?
  A. perineum
  B. perimetrium
  C. myometrium
  D. endometrium

_C_ **25.** The largest layer of the uterus is the
  A. perineum
  B. perimetrium
  C. myometrium
  D. endometrium

_A_ **26.** The upper openings of the uterine cavity join with the
  A. fallopian tubes
  B. cervical canal
  C. fimbriae
  D. external os

_B_ **27.** The lower opening of the uterine cavity joins with the
  A. fallopian tubes
  B. cervical canal
  C. fimbriae
  D. external os

_D_ **28.** The upper opening of the cervical canal is called the
  A. cilia
  B. external os
  C. fimbriae
  D. internal os

_B_ **29.** The lower opening of the cervical canal is called the
  A. cilia
  B. external os
  C. fimbriae
  D. internal os

_C_ **30.** The organ in which the fetus develops and grows and from which it is expelled at birth is the
  A. pelvis
  B. vagina
  C. uterus
  D. ovary

_D_ **31.** The ovum is received by and assisted to the uterus by means of the
  (1) fimbriated ends of the fallopian tubes
  (2) wavelike movements of the cilia
  (3) peristaltic action of the fallopian tubes
  (4) ovarian ligaments
  A. All of these
  B. (1) and (2)
  C. (2), (3), and (4)
  D. (1), (2), and (3)

_A_ **32.** The female sex glands are called
  A. ovaries
  B. primary follicles
  C. graafian follicle
  D. pituitary

_C_ **33.** Once a month, from puberty until menopause, a graafian follicle ruptures and expels a mature ovum. This process is called
  A. menstruation
  B. proliferative phase
  C. ovulation
  D. secretory phase

_D_ **34.** Hormones produced by the female sex gland are
(1) follicle-stimulating hormone
(2) progesterone
(3) luteinizing hormone
(4) estrogen
A. (1) and (2)
B. (2) and (3)
C. (3) and (4)
D. (2) and (4)
E. (1) and (3)

_D_ **35.** The female sex hormone is
A. follicle-stimulating hormone
B. progesterone
C. luteinizing hormone
D. estrogen

_A_ **36.** Ovulation usually occurs about
A. 14 days before the beginning of the next menstrual period
B. 14 days after the beginning of the last menstrual period
C. 7 days before the beginning of the next menstrual period
D. 7 days after the beginning of the last menstrual period

_B_ **37.** Which of the following is *not* a function of progesterone?
A. It prepares the endometrium for pregnancy
B. It is responsible for the development of the distinctive female characteristics
C. It maintains the endometrium during pregnancy
D. It suppresses ovulation during pregnancy

_D_ **38.** Hormonal control of the menstrual cycle is initiated by the
A. thyroid gland
B. ovaries
C. corpus luteum
D. pituitary gland

_A_ **39.** In order for pregnancy to occur, following ovulation the ovum must be fertilized within
A. 48 hours
B. 24 hours
C. 3 to 4 days
D. 6 to 8 days

_D_ **40.** Following fertilization, the length of time it takes for the fertilized ovum to become imbedded in the endometrium is
A. 48 hours
B. 24 hours
C. 3 to 4 days
D. 6 to 8 days

_A_ **41.** A woman who is keeping a basal temperature record to find out when she ovulates needs to know that, usually,
(1) a drop in temperature immediately precedes ovulation
(2) a drop in temperature follows ovulation
(3) a rise in temperature immediately precedes ovulation
(4) a rise in temperature follows ovulation
A. (1) and (4)
B. (2) and (3)
C. (1) only
D. (3) only

_C_ **42.** Which of the following is *not* a part of the true pelvis?
A. inlet
B. cavity
C. ilium
D. outlet

_C_ **43.** Which of the following are *not* located within the cavity of the true pelvis?
A. urinary bladder
B. rectum
C. mammary glands
D. internal female reproductive organs

44. The false pelvis is important in obstetrics because
    (1) it supports the growing uterus during pregnancy
    (2) it directs the fetus into the true pelvis near the end of pregnancy
    (3) by determining its size, the doctor may be able to estimate the size of the true pelvis
    (4) it is the organ which nourishes the growing fetus
    A. All of these
    B. All except (3)
    C. All except (2)
    D. All except (4)

45. The true pelvis is important in obstetrics because
    A. the baby must pass through it to be born
    B. it supports the growing uterus during pregnancy
    C. it is the organ which nourishes the growing fetus
    D. it contains all the female organs of reproduction

46. Which of the following are important differences between the female pelvis and the male pelvis?
    (1) The inlet, cavity, and outlet of the true pelvis are larger in the female pelvis than in the male
    (2) The pubic arch is wider and the coccyx is more movable in the female pelvis than in the male
    (3) The pubic arch is narrower and the coccyx is less movable in the female pelvis than in the male
    (4) The inlet, cavity, and outlet of the true pelvis are smaller in the female pelvis than in the male
    A. (1) and (3)
    B. (2) and (4)
    C. (3) and (4)
    D. (1) and (2)

47. Which of the following are *not* female reproductive organs but are functionally or anatomically related to them?
    (1) mammary glands
    (2) urinary bladder
    (3) gallbladder
    (4) rectum
    A. (1) only
    B. (3) only
    C. (1), (2), and (4)
    D. (1), (3), and (4)

48. The external male reproductive organs consist of the
    A. prostate gland and Cowper's glands
    B. testes and epididymis
    C. vans deferens and ejaculatory duct
    D. penis and scrotum

49. Circumcision is the surgical removal of the
    A. glans penis
    B. foreskin of the penis
    C. scrotum
    D. vas deferens

50. Spermatozoa are produced by the
    A. penis
    B. testes
    C. epididymis
    D. prostate gland

51. The male sex hormone is produced by the
    A. seminal vesicles
    B. cells of Leydig
    C. Cowper's glands
    D. prostate gland

52. Compared to ova, spermatozoa are
    A. much smaller
    B. a little smaller
    C. much larger
    D. a little larger

_D_ **53.** Which of the following are canals or tubes through which the spermatozoa pass as they are transported to the outside of the body?
   (1) epididymis
   (2) vas deferens
   (3) ejaculatory duct
   (4) urethra
   A. (2) only
   B. All except (4)
   C. (1) and (2)
   D. All of these

_B_ **54.** Which of the following does *not* produce secretions which provide a fluid medium in which spermatozoa are sustained and transported?
   A. seminal vesicles
   B. seminiferous tubules
   C. prostate gland
   D. bulbourethral glands

_A_ **55.** Prostate secretions are
   A. thin and alkaline
   B. thick and acid
   C. thick and alkaline
   D. thin and acid

_C_ **56.** Sperm motility is greatest in
   A. acid media
   B. alkaline media
   C. neutral or slightly alkaline media
   D. neutral or slightly acid media

_D_ **57.** The number of spermatozoa deposited in the vagina at each ejaculation is
   A. one
   B. about 300
   C. about 300 thousand
   D. about 300 million

_A_ **58.** The number of spermatozoa which penetrates, and thereby fertilizes, the ovum is
   A. one
   B. about 300
   C. about 300 thousand
   D. about 300 million

_A_ **59.** Once the sperm enters the female reproductive tract, it may be capable of fertilizing the ovum for
   A. hours or days
   B. less than an hour
   C. more than a week
   D. a month

_D_ **60.** Probably the most complicated to use and the least effective of the contraceptive methods is the
   A. condom
   B. pill
   C. diaphragm
   D. rhythm method

_B_ **61.** When a couple decides they definitely do not want any more children, permanent sterilization of the woman can be accomplished by
   (1) vasectomy
   (2) hysterectomy
   (3) tubal ligation
   (4) coitus interruptus
   A. (1) only
   B. (2) and (3)
   C. (4) only
   D. (1) and (4)

_A_ **62.** Sterilization of the man can be accomplished by
   A. vasectomy
   B. hysterectomy
   C. tubal ligation
   D. coitus interruptus

_C_ **63.** As a result of high technology the options available to infertile couples today include
  (1) surrogate embryo transfer
  (2) in vitro fertilization and embryo transfer
  (3) gamete intrafallopian transfer
  (4) artificial insemination
  (5) adoption of children
  A. (4) and (5)
  B. (2), (3),and (5)
  C. (1), (2),and (3)
  D. All of these

_D_ **64.** Which of the following would the infertile couple be _least_ likely to experience?
  A. frustration
  B. isolation
  C. low self-esteem
  D. high self-esteem

III. Diagram and explain the hormonal control of the normal menstrual cycle.

IV. Prepare a nursing care plan for an infertile couple.

ASSESSMENTS	POTENTIAL NURSING DIAGNOSES	INTERVENTIONS	EXPECTED OUTCOMES

ANSWERS · CHAPTER 5

I. **A.** Mons pubis **E.** Perineum
B. Clitoris **F.** Labium major
C. Urethra **G.** Labium minor
D. Vagina **H.** Anus

II.

1. B	**17.** A	**33.** C	**49.** B
2. D	**18.** D	**34.** D	**50.** B
3. C	**19.** C	**35.** D	**51.** B
4. A	**20.** C	**36.** A	**52.** A
5. C	**21.** A	**37.** B	**53.** D
6. A	**22.** A	**38.** D	**54.** B
7. D	**23.** D	**39.** A	**55.** A
8. B	**24.** A	**40.** D	**56.** C
9. A	**25.** C	**41.** A	**57.** D
10. C	**26.** A	**42.** C	**58.** A
11. B	**27.** B	**43.** C	**59.** A
12. B	**28.** D	**44.** D	**60.** D
13. A	**29.** B	**45.** A	**61.** B
14. B	**30.** C	**46.** D	**62.** A
15. D	**31.** D	**47.** C	**63.** C
16. C	**32.** A	**48.** D	**64.** D

III. Hormonal control of the normal menstrual cycle.

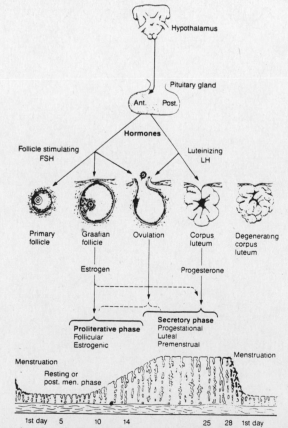

IV. See Chapter 5 of *Introductory Maternity Nursing,* 5th edition.

description and effects 6 of pregnancy

I. SITUATION: Before they were married, Debbie and Bob discussed their feelings and desires concerning a family. They agreed that, although they each loved children and would like to have two or three, they wanted to wait until they were able to do so without financial strain. Consequently, for the first 4 years of their marriage, Debbie took birth control pills. In March she stopped taking the pill. She had regular menstrual periods beginning on April 11, May 9, and June 6. In July she missed a period. When she did not have a period by the middle of August she went to the doctor to see if she was pregnant. He did an antigen-antibody test and it was positive.

Place the letter of the *best* answer in the space before the statement.

C___ **1.** With this pregnancy, Debbie is a
   A. multipara
   B. multigravida
   C. primigravida
   D. para I, gravida 0

C___ **2.** Using the five digit system, with this pregnancy Debbie would be a gravida
   A. 1-0-0-1-0
   B. 0-1-0-0-0
   C. 1-0-0-0-0
   D. 1-0-0-0-1

B___ **3.** Using Naegele's rule, Debbie's estimated date of confinement is
   A. February 6
   B. March 13
   C. April 13
   D. April 6

A___ **4.** The number of days in a lunar month is
   A. 28
   B. 280
   C. 30
   D. 300

D___ **5.** The length of a full-term pregnancy in weeks is
   A. 28
   B. 280
   C. 10
   D. 40

A___ **6.** Another term for birth is
   A. parturition
   B. conception
   C. gestation
   D. gravida

D___ **7.** The medical term for a pregnant woman is
   A. parturition
   B. conception
   C. gestation
   D. gravida

_C_ **8.** Another term for pregnancy is
  A. parturition
  B. conception
  C. gestation
  D. gravida

_A_ **9.** During the first 5 weeks of pregnancy, the developing organism is called
  A. embryo
  B. fetus
  C. nullipara
  D. abortion

_B_ **10.** After the first 5 weeks of pregnancy, the developing organism is called
  A. embryo
  B. fetus
  C. nullipara
  D. abortion

_C_ **11.** The term "viable" or "age of viability" when applied to pregnancy means the pregnancy has progressed to the point where the fetus is
  A. dead
  B. alive
  C. capable of surviving outside the uterus
  D. incapable of surviving outside the uterus

_B_ **12.** The term that applies to previous pregnancies that terminated after the age of viability is
  A. gravida
  B. para
  C. abortion
  D. premature labor

_A_ **13.** A pregnancy that terminates before the age of viability is called
  A. abortion
  B. premature labor
  C. trimester
  D. term pregnancy

_B_ **14.** A pregnancy that ends after the age of viability but before full term is called
  A. abortion
  B. premature labor
  C. trimester
  D. term pregnancy

_C_ **15.** Pregnancy is divided into 3-month periods called
  A. lunar months
  B. calendar months
  C. trimesters
  D. parturition

_A_ **16.** Naegele's rule is used to calculate the estimated date of
  A. delivery
  B. conception
  C. viability
  D. ovulation

_B_ **17.** In order to use Naegele's rule, one must know
  A. the first day of the patient's last ovulation
  B. the first day of the patient's last menstrual period
  C. the last day of the patient's last ovulation
  D. the last day of the patient's last menstrual period

_D_ **18.** One of the presumptive signs Debbie is likely to be aware of early in pregnancy is
  A. quickening
  B. Braxton Hicks contractions
  C. enlargement of the abdomen
  D. amenorrhea

_C_ **19.** Nausea and vomiting during pregnancy usually occurs between the
  A. first and fourth weeks
  B. fourth and eighth weeks
  C. fourth and twelfth weeks
  D. fourth and sixteenth weeks

_C_   **20.** Theories regarding the cause of morning sickness attribute it to
  (1) subconscious rejection of the pregnancy
  (2) changes in carbohydrate metabolism
  (3) an increase in hormones
  (4) subconscious hunger
  A. (1) and (2)
  B. (3) and (4)
  C. All except (4)
  D. the cause is not known

_A_   **21.** Certain of the probable signs of pregnancy are due to the increased blood supply and increased hormones produced during pregnancy. Which of the following is *not* caused by these?
  A. Braxton Hicks contractions
  B. Chadwick's sign
  C. Goodell's sign
  D. Hegar's sign

_C_   **22.** Most pregnancy tests are based on the presence of a certain hormone in the blood or urine of the woman. The hormone is
  A. estrogen
  B. progesterone
  C. chorionic gonadotropin
  D. chorionic villi

_D_   **23.** In obtaining a urine specimen for a pregnancy test the nurse should
  (1) catheterize the patient
  (2) instruct the patient to avoid drinking fluids after the evening meal the night before the test
  (3) obtain the first voided specimen in the morning
  (4) refrigerate the urine until the test is done
  A. All except (3)
  B. (1) only
  C. (3) only
  D. All except (1)

II. In the space before each sign of pregnancy in Column I, place the letter from Column II that indicates whether it is a presumptive, probable, or positive sign of pregnancy.

Page 96

	I SIGN OF PREGNANCY	II TYPE OF SIGN
_B_	**1.** Fetal outline by palpation	**A.** Presumptive sign
_C_	**2.** Fetal outline by ultrasound or x-ray	**B.** Probable sign
_B_	**3.** Braxton Hicks contractions	**C.** Positive sign
_A_	**4.** Breast changes	
_A_	**5.** Amenorrhea	
_B_	**6.** Enlargement of the abdomen	
_A_	**7.** Pigmentation	
_A_	**8.** Chadwick's sign	
_B_	**9.** Goodell's sign	
_C_	**10.** Hearing fetal heartbeat	
_A_	**11.** Quickening	
_C_	**12.** Fetal movement felt by examiner	
_B_	**13.** Ballottement	
_A_	**14.** Frequency of urination	
_B_	**15.** Positive pregnancy tests	
_A_	**16.** Nausea and vomiting	
_B_	**17.** Hegar's sign	

III. DISCUSSION: Write a paragraph describing how each of the following might react initially to being told by her doctor that she is pregnant.

1. A woman who has had an infertility problem

2. A 42-year-old woman who has two grandchildren and whose youngest child is 15 years old

3. An unmarried teenager

IV. SITUATION: Since Debbie and Bob are expecting their first child, they are interested in learning as much as they can about pregnancy and the changes it produces. You help them by explaining how pregnancy affects the reproductive system and other parts of the body.

Place the letter of the *best* answer in the space before the statement.

_B_ **1.** The most marked changes in the body resulting from pregnancy occur in the
  A. breasts
  B. uterus
  C. circulatory system
  D. nervous system

_D_ **2.** The size of the uterus increases from approximately 1 inch deep × 2 inches wide × 3 inches long to
  A. 12 to 14 inches deep × 8 to 10 inches wide × 8 to 9 inches long
  B. 12 to 14 inches wide × 8 to 10 inches long × 8 to 9 inches deep
  C. 12 to 14 inches long × 8 to 10 inches deep × 8 to 9 inches wide
  D. 12 to 14 inches long × 8 to 10 inches wide × 8 to 9 inches deep

_A_ **3.** The weight of the uterus increases from about 2 oz to
   A. 2 lb
   B. 3 lb
   C. 1 lb
   D. 4 lb

_D_ **4.** During pregnancy the capacity of the uterus increases more than
   A. 200 times
   B. 300 times
   C. 400 times
   D. 500 times

_A_ **5.** The increased size of the uterus during pregnancy is attributed to
   (1) growth of the muscle fibers
   (2) development of new muscle cells
   (3) hormone stimulation and increased blood supply
   (4) growth of the fetus
   A. All of these
   B. All except (4)
   C. (2) only
   D. (1) and (3)

_A_ **6.** During pregnancy the cervix becomes
   A. shorter and softer
   B. longer and softer
   C. shorter and harder
   D. longer and harder

_C_ **7.** During pregnancy the number of muscle cells in the cervix
   A. increases and those that were there decrease in size
   B. increases and those that were there increase in size
   C. decreases and those that remain increase in size
   D. decreases and those that remain decrease in size

_D_ **8.** The secretions from the cervical glands form a mucus plug in the cervical canal. This mucus plug
   A. causes softening of the cervix
   B. prevents effacement of the cervical canal
   C. prevents dilatation of the os
   D. acts as a barrier against infection

_C_ **9.** During pregnancy, changes that occur in the ovaries and fallopian tubes include:
   (1) new follicles do not mature
   (2) ovulation continues
   (3) ovulation ceases
   (4) the ovaries and tubes change from a vertical to a horizontal position
   A. All except (3)
   B. (1), (3), and (4)
   C. (1) and (3)
   D. (2) and (4)

_C_ **10.** The following are all changes which occur in the vagina during pregnancy. Which one is the most likely to cause Debbie discomfort?
   A. increased blood supply and hypertrophy of the muscle cells
   B. bluish or purplish discoloration
   C. increased vaginal secretions
   D. thickening of the mucosa and loosening of the connective tissue

_B_ **11.** Some of the changes which occur in the vagina help prepare it for the birth of the baby. These include
   (1) increased blood supply and hypertrophy of the muscle cells
   (2) bluish or purplish discoloration
   (3) increased vaginal secretions
   (4) thickening of the mucosa and loosening of the connective tissue
   A. (1) and (2)
   B. (1) and (4)
   C. (2) and (3)
   D. (2) and (4)

_A_ **12.** You can tell Debbie that the changes that occur in the breasts during pregnancy
   (1) are due to hormonal stimulation
   (2) prepare them for lactation
   (3) may cause striae gravidarum
   (4) bring about production of colostrum
   A. All of these
   B. All except (3)
   C. (2) and (4)
   D. (1) and (2)

_A_ **13.** Which of the following is *not* a change in the pelvis during pregnancy?
   A. decreased mobility of the pelvic bones
   B. increased blood supply and hormonal activity
   C. relaxation of the pelvic joints
   D. increased mobility of the pelvic bones

_D_ **14.** The backache experienced by Debbie during pregnancy may be due to
   (1) decreased mobility of the pelvic bones
   (2) increased blood supply and hormonal activity
   (3) relaxation of the pelvic joints
   (4) shifting the weight of the uterus to the surrounding muscles and ligaments
   A. (1) only
   B. (1) and (3)
   C. (1), (2), and (4)
   D. (2), (3), and (4)

_C_ **15.** During pregnancy, Debbie can expect her blood volume to
   A. increase about 50%
   B. decrease about 50%
   C. increase about 30%
   D. decrease about 30%

_C_ **16.** In order to meet the needs of herself and her unborn baby, Debbie should maintain a hemoglobin of at least
   A. 10 g and a hematocrit of 30%
   B. 8 g and a hematocrit of 24%
   C. 12 g and a hematocrit of 35%
   D. 20 g and a hematocrit of 60%

_A_ **17.** Debbie's blood pressure before pregnancy was normal. During normal pregnancy she can expect it to
   A. remain normal
   B. drop considerably
   C. increase slightly
   D. increase considerably

_C_ **18.** During the latter part of pregnancy, Debbie may experience some discomforts resulting from the pressure of the uterus on the pelvic veins. Which of the following is *not* one of these discomforts?
   A. hemorrhoids
   B. varicose veins
   C. shortness of breath
   D. edema of her feet and ankles

_B_ **19.** Bob tells you that recently Debbie has complained about her gums bleeding when she brushes her teeth. You can explain that this is probably due to
   A. decreased gastric motility
   B. large amounts of estrogen in her body
   C. increased blood supply
   D. decreased hormones

_A_ **20.** Debbie eats a well-balanced diet and was in excellent health when she became pregnant. You would consider a desirable weight gain for her to be about
   A. 25 to 30 lb
   B. 34 to 37 lb
   C. 10 to 15 lb
   D. 15 to 20 lb

_D_ **21.** The weight Debbie gains during pregnancy can be attributed to each of the following. However, she may have most difficulty losing the weight gained through
   A. growth of her reproductive organs
   B. growth of the products of conception
   C. retention of fluid in her tissues and blood
   D. deposits of fat

_B_ **22.** Stretch marks which may appear on Debbie's breasts, abdomen, thighs, or buttocks are called
   A. chloasma
   B. striae gravidarum
   C. linea nigra
   D. diastasis recti

_A_ **23.** You can tell Debbie that the irregular, patchy pigmentation on her face is called the "mask of pregnancy." Another name for it is
   A. chloasma
   B. striae gravidarum
   C. linea nigra
   D. diastasis recti

_C_ **24.** She asks you if she will always have this "horrid mask of pregnancy." You can answer that, after the baby is born, it will
   A. become lighter
   B. become darker
   C. disappear completely
   D. have to be surgically removed

_B_ **25.** Debbie also asks what will happen to her stretch marks. You can reply that, after the baby is born, they will
   A. disappear completely
   B. become silvery in appearance
   C. become redder
   D. have to be surgically removed

V. In the space before the discomfort in Column I, place the letter or letters of the probable cause from Column II.

I	II
DISCOMFORT	**PROBABLE CAUSE**

_G_   **1.** Heartburn   **A.** Pelvic bone mobility

_DI_   **2.** Hoarse voice   **B.** Pressure from uterus on pelvic veins

_B_   **3.** Varicose veins   **C.** Pressure from uterus on bladder

_F_   **4.** Shortness of breath   **D.** Increased blood supply

_J_   **5.** Constipation   **E.** Large amounts of estrogen in the body

_G_   **6.** Flatulence   **F.** Pressure of uterus on diaphragm

_G_   **7.** Vomiting   **G.** Decreased gastric motility

_C_   **8.** Frequency of urination   **H.** Dilatation of ureters and statis of urine

_HI_   **9.** Urinary tract infections   **I.** Increased hormonal activity

_B_   **10.** Hemorrhoids   **J.** Loss of tone of gastrointestinal tract

_A_   **11.** Waddly gait

_DI_   **12.** Nosebleeds

_E_   **13.** Ptyalism

_B_   **14.** Edema of ankles and feet

I.
1. C	7. D	13. A	19. C
2. C	8. C	14. B	20. C
3. B	9. A	15. C	21. A
4. A	10. B	16. A	22. C
5. D	11. C	17. B	23. D
6. A	12. B	18. D	

II.
1. B	6. B	11. A	16. A
2. C	7. A	12. C	17. B
3. B	8. B	13. B	
4. A	9. B	14. A	
5. A	10. C	15. B	

III. See Chapter 6 of *Introductory Maternity Nursing,* 5th edition.

IV.
1. B	8. D	15. C	22. B
2. D	9. C	16. C	23. A
3. A	10. C	17. A	24. C
4. D	11. B	18. C	25. B
5. A	12. A	19. B	
6. A	13. A	20. A	
7. C	14. D	21. D	

V.
1. G	5. J	9. H, I	13. E
2. D, I	6. G	10. B	14. B
3. B	7. G	11. A	
4. F	8. C	12. D, I	

fetal development 7

I. Place the letter of the *best* answer in the space before the statement.

1. The two types of cells in the human body are
A. ova and sperm
B. chromosomes and genes
C. gamete and zygote
D. soma and germ

2. Sex cells do not mature and are not capable of functioning until
A. maturation
B. puberty
C. conception
D. ovulation

3. The total number of chromosomes in each body cell in human beings is
A. 46
B. 48
C. 23
D. 96

4. During maturation, the number of chromosomes in each sex cell is reduced to
A. 46
B. 48
C. 23
D. 24

5. A mature sex cell is called a
A. zygote
B. gamete
C. gene
D. chromosome

6. When a mature sex cell from the male and a mature sex cell from the female unite, the new cell formed is called a
A. zygote
B. gamete
C. gene
D. chromosome

7. The factors responsible for the characteristics or traits of individuals are carried by
A. zygotes
B. gametes
C. genes
D. chromosomes

8. All inherited characteristics and traits are determined at
A. maturation
B. puberty
C. ovulation
D. conception

_B_ 9. The sex of each individual is determined at
   A. puberty
   B. conception
   C. ovulation
   D. maturation

_A_ 10. Fertilization usually occurs in the
   A. fallopian tube
   B. ovary
   C. uterus
   D. vagina

_D_ 11. Following fertilization, while the ovum is traveling toward the uterus, it becomes a mass of cells called a
   A. trophoblast
   B. blastocyst
   C. villi
   D. morula

_A_ 12. After the cells divide into two layers, the outer layer obtains food for the inner layer. The outer layer is called the
   A. trophoblast
   B. blastocyst
   C. villi
   D. morula

_D_ 13. Following fertilization, the journey of the ovum to the uterus usually takes
   A. 2 to 3 hours
   B. 2 to 3 days
   C. 3 to 6 hours
   D. 3 to 6 days

_B_ 14. After the fertilized ovum reaches the uterus, the length of time before it begins to embed itself in the lining of the uterine cavity is
   A. 2 to 3 hours
   B. 2 to 3 days
   C. 3 to 6 hours
   D. 3 to 6 days

_C_ 15. During pregnancy the lining of the uterine cavity is called the
   A. endometrium
   B. chorion
   C. decidua
   D. amnion

_B_ 16. The rootlike projections on the chorion which contain blood vessels connected to the fetus are called
   A. amnion
   B. villi
   C. decidua
   D. trophoblast

_B_ 17. Soon after implantation, two membranes form around the embryo. The outer membrane is the
   A. amnion
   B. chorion
   C. decidua
   D. placenta

_A_ 18. The inner membrane which forms around the embryo is the
   A. amnion
   B. chorion
   C. decidua
   D. placenta

_B_ 19. Which of the following is *not* a function of the amniotic fluid?
   A. protects fetus from injury
   B. provides oxygen and rids fetus of waste products
   C. provides a constant temperature for fetus
   D. permits fetus to move about freely

_A_   **20.** The average amount of amniotic fluid present at term is
       A. 1 liter
       B. 2 liters
       C. 300 ml
       D. 100 ml

_A_   **21.** Which of the following is *not* one of the three germ layers from which specific structures develop?
       A. perioderm
       B. ectoderm
       C. mesoderm
       D. entoderm

_C_   **22.** The structure that supplies oxygen and nourishment to the fetus, and through which its waste products are eliminated, is the
       A. amniotic fluid
       B. chorion
       C. placenta
       D. decidua

_B_   **23.** The placenta is usually developed by the end of the
       A. first week after fertilization
       B. first month after fertilization
       C. third week after fertilization
       D. third month after fertilization

_B_   **24.** Transfer of oxygen and nourishment for the fetus and the elimination of waste products by the fetus occur through the process of
       A. diffusion
       B. osmosis
       C. precipitation
       D. agglutination

_A_   **25.** The maternal side of the placenta is composed of 15 to 20 segments called
       A. cotyledons
       B. membranes
       C. umbilical cord
       D. Wharton's jelly

_D_   **26.** During the second and third trimesters of pregnancy, the "placental barrier" is made up of
       A. four layers of cells
       B. three layers of cells
       C. two layers of cells
       D. one layer of cells

_C_   **27.** The connecting link between the fetus and the placenta is the
       A. cotyledons
       B. membranes
       C. umbilical cord
       D. amnion

_B_   **28.** The umbilical cord contains
       A. one artery and two veins
       B. one vein and two arteries
       C. two veins and two arteries
       D. one vein and one artery

_D_   **29.** At term, the umbilical cord is usually about
       A. 10 to 12 inches long
       B. 14 to 16 inches long
       C. 18 to 20 inches long
       D. 20 to 22 inches long

_A_   **30.** The vessels in the umbilical cord are surrounded and protected by
       A. Wharton's jelly
       B. membranes
       C. amniotic fluid
       D. cotyledons

_C_   **31.** Which of the following is not a hormone produced by the placenta?
       A. chorionic gonadotropin
       B. estrogen
       C. lactogen
       D. progesterone

_B_ **32.** Fetal circulation differs from circulation after birth because the
  A. fetus does not need as much blood before birth
  B. fetal lungs do not function before birth
  C. fetal liver does not function before birth
  D. fetal heart does not function before birth

_B_ **33.** Which of the following is *not* one of the structures in fetal circulation which disappears after birth?
  A. ductus venosus
  B. inferior vena cava
  C. ductus arteriosus
  D. foramen ovale

_A_ **34.** Identical twins develop from
  A. one ovum fertilized by one sperm
  B. one ovum fertilized by two sperm
  C. two ova fertilized by two sperm
  D. two ova fertilized by one sperm

_C_ **35.** Fraternal twins develop from
  A. one ovum fertilized by one sperm
  B. one ovum fertilized by two sperm
  C. two ova fertilized by two sperm
  D. two ova fertilized by one sperm

II. Underline the correct word or phrase in parentheses that will make the statement true.

1. After maturation, the ovum always contains (an **X** chromosome, a **Y** chromosome).
2. When a sperm containing an **X** chromosome unites with an ovum, the child will be a (girl, boy).
3. When a sperm containing a **Y** chromosome unites with an ovum, the child will be a (girl, boy).
4. The sex of the new individual is determined by the (mother, father).
5. Each time a sperm unites with an ovum there is a (40–60, 50–50) chance that the child will be a girl and a (60–40, 50–50) chance that it will be a boy.
6. The fetal side of the placenta is (rough and irregular, smooth and shiny).
7. The umbilical cord is attached to the (fetal side, maternal side) of the placenta.
8. The oxygenated blood for the fetus is carried through the (vein, arteries) of the umbilical cord.
9. The waste products of the fetus are eliminated through the (vein, arteries) of the umbilical cord.
10. Before birth, the fetus lives in a (lower, higher) oxygen concentration than after birth.

III. In the space before the stage of development in Column I, place the letter of the period of gestation from Column II that tells when it first is present. (Each phase of development is completed at the end of the period given.)

I	II
STAGE OF DEVELOPMENT	**PERIOD OF GESTATION**

_D_ **1.** Sex of fetus obvious   **A.** first lunar month
_I_ **2.** Chance of survival excellent   **B.** second lunar month
_E_ **3.** Lanugo present   **C.** third lunar month
_C_ **4.** Teeth forming under the gums   **D.** fourth lunar month
_F_ **5.** Vernix caseosa present   **E.** fifth lunar month
_E_ **6.** Quickening   **F.** sixth lunar month
_D_ **7.** Meconium   **G.** seventh lunar month
_C_ **8.** Centers of ossification appear in most bones   **H.** eighth lunar month
_E_ **9.** Hair on the head   **I.** ninth lunar month
_J_ **10.** Fetus mature   **J.** tenth lunar month
_A_ **11.** All organs present in rudimentary form

ANSWERS · CHAPTER 7

I.
1. D
2. B
3. A
4. C
5. B
6. A
7. C
8. D
9. B
10. A
11. D
12. A
13. D
14. B
15. C
16. B
17. B
18. A
19. B
20. A
21. A
22. C
23. B
24. B
25. A
26. D
27. C
28. B
29. D
30. A
31. C
32. B
33. B
34. A
35. C

II.
1. an **X** chromosome
2. girl
3. boy
4. father
5. 50–50, 50–50
6. smooth and shiny
7. fetal side
8. vein
9. arteries
10. lower

III.
1. D
2. I
3. E
4. C
5. F
6. E
7. D
8. C
9. E
10. J
11. A

health care during **8** pregnancy

I. SITUATION: Debbie and Bob are from homes with strong family ties where children are loved and wanted. As an intelligent, well-educated couple, they recognize the importance of medical supervision to a happy outcome to pregnancy. Therefore, as soon as they suspected that Debbie might be pregnant, they made an appointment with an obstetrician.

Place the letter of the *best* answer in the space before the statement.

_A_ **1.** The health care Debbie receives during her pregnancy is called
   A. antepartal care
   B. intrapartal care
   C. postpartal care
   D. none of these

_C_ **2.** Prenatal, or antepartal, care was first begun by
   A. obstetricians
   B. midwives
   C. nurses
   D. family practice physicians

_D_ **3.** Debbie can expect that the care she receives will include
   (1) evaluating her health status
   (2) correcting any existing health problems
   (3) preventing health problems
   (4) promoting positive health
   A. (1) and (2)
   B. (2) and (4)
   C. (2) and (3)
   D. All of these

_B_ **4.** Which of the following potential nursing diagnoses for a pregnant woman is *least* likely to be appropriate for Debbie?
   A. alteration in comfort related to normal body changes during pregnancy
   B. alteration in nutrition, less than needed for pregnancy and the developing fetus
   C. knowledge deficit related to the procedures performed in the doctor's office
   D. anxiety related to exposure of her body during examinations and procedures

_A_ **5.** To ensure adequate medical supervision during pregnancy, Debbie should visit her doctor at least
   A. monthly until the seventh month, then every 2 weeks until the last month, and then every week until the baby is born
   B. every 2 weeks until the seventh month, then every week until the baby is born
   C. every 2 months until the seventh month, then every month until the baby is born
   D. every month until the eighth month, then every 2 weeks until the baby is born

_C_ **6.** A balanced diet during pregnancy consists of the daily intake of
   (1) 1 quart of milk
   (2) four or more servings of bread and cereals
   (3) two or more servings of meat, fish, eggs, or cheese
   (4) four or more servings of vegetables and fruits
   A. All except (2)
   B. (1) and (3)
   C. All of these
   D. (3) and (4)

_D_ **7.** Debbie normally eats a balanced diet. Therefore, the only changes she needs to make in her diet are to increase her intake of foods containing
   (1) minerals
   (2) vitamins
   (3) proteins
   (4) carbohydrates
   A. All of these
   B. All except (2)
   C. All except (3)
   D. All except (4)

_B_ **8.** Which of the following is *not* a mineral that Debbie needs to increase in her diet during pregnancy?
   A. phosphorus
   B. sodium
   C. calcium
   D. iron

_C_ **9.** During pregnancy, Debbie's daily intake of calcium should be
   A. 0.5 g
   B. 1.0 g
   C. 1.2 g
   D. 2 g

_B_ **10.** Calcium and phosphorus are essential components of bones and teeth. In addition, calcium is necessary for
   (1) the formation of hemoglobin
   (2) normal contractility of muscles
   (3) maintenance of the heartbeat
   (4) normal clotting of the blood
   A. All of these
   B. All except (1)
   C. All except (4)
   D. (2) and (3)

_A_ **11.** Debbie should know that the best source of calcium is
   A. milk
   B. cheese
   C. green, leafy vegetables
   D. meat

_D_ **12.** Debbie should include additional iron in her diet during pregnancy because iron is necessary for
   (1) formation of hemoglobin
   (2) transporting oxygen and carbon dioxide
   (3) normal contractility of muscles
   (4) maintenance of the heartbeat
   A. All of these
   B. (2) and (3)
   C. (1) and (4)
   D. (1) and (2)

_D_ **13.** Because its diet for a while after birth is poor in iron, the fetus stores up iron during
   A. all of pregnancy
   B. the first trimester
   C. the second trimester
   D. the last trimester

_A_ **14.** This supply of iron should be adequate for
   A. 5 months
   B. 5 weeks
   C. 2 months
   D. 1 month

_C_ **15.** Debbie especially needs to increase her intake of vitamin
   (1) A
   (2) E
   (3) C
   (4) D
   A. All of these
   B. All except (1)
   C. All except (2)
   D. All except (4)

_A_ **16.** Which of these vitamins does not cross the placental barrier?
- **A.** A
- **B.** E
- **C.** C
- **D.** D

_A_ **17.** Which of these vitamins is obtained by the breast-fed infant through the colostrum and breast milk?
- **A.** A
- **B.** E
- **C.** C
- **D.** D

_C_ **18.** Which of the following is *not* a function of vitamin C?
- **A.** helps make the blood vessel walls
- **B.** aids in the healing of wounds
- **C.** is essential for the absorption and utilization of calcium
- **D.** is necessary for the development of normal connective tissue

_C_ **19.** Which of the following would be a better source of protein than of vitamins?
- **A.** dark green, leafy vegetables
- **B.** tomatoes
- **C.** lean meat
- **D.** fresh fruit

_B_ **20.** Debbie should increase her daily intake of protein by about
- **A.** 5 g
- **B.** 30 g
- **C.** 100 g
- **D.** 15 g

_A_ **21.** Debbie needs additional protein during pregnancy because it is
- **(1)** necessary for the development of the new muscles in the uterus
- **(2)** essential to the formation, growth, and development of the embryo
- **(3)** needed for the manufacture of hormones
- **(4)** a constituent of blood
- **A.** All of these
- **B.** All except (1)
- **C.** All except (4)
- **D.** (2) and (3)

_C_ **22.** In choosing her maternity wardrobe, it would be well for Debbie to remember that
- **(1)** her clothing should not constrict her blood vessels
- **(2)** her clothing should allow for expansion of her growing uterus
- **(3)** her bras should have wide straps and give support without pressure
- **(4)** she should always wear a girdle or corset
- **A.** (1), (2), and (4)
- **B.** (2), (3), and (4)
- **C.** (1), (2), and (3)
- **D.** (1), (3), and (4)

_D_ **23.** In choosing her shoes, she should remember that
- **(1)** they should provide good support
- **(2)** shoes with high heels may exaggerate the swayback posture of pregnancy
- **(3)** shoes with broad heels may help prevent falls
- **(4)** shoes with broad heels may help prevent backache
- **A.** All except (2)
- **B.** (1) and (2)
- **C.** (3) and (4)
- **D.** All of these

_B_ **24.** One of the best exercises for Debbie during pregnancy is
- **A.** playing tennis
- **B.** brisk walking in the fresh air
- **C.** jogging
- **D.** swimming

_A_ **25.** In her job at the bank it is necessary for Debbie to sit for long periods at a time. Now that she is pregnant she should
- **A.** have frequent rest periods when she can change her position and elevate her legs for a few minutes
- **B.** quit working until after the baby is born
- **C.** work fewer hours each day
- **D.** change to another job that does not require sitting for long periods of time

26. Now that she is pregnant Debbie should
  (1) take showers, never a tub bath
  (2) take tub baths, never a shower
  (3) take a tub bath or shower as she wishes
  (4) be very careful when getting in and out of the tub so as to avoid falling
  A. (1) only
  B. (2) only
  C. (3) only
  D. (3) and (4)

27. Since Debbie plans to breast-feed her baby, you can suggest ways of helping her prepare her nipples. These would include
  (1) daily cleansing with a washcloth and warm water
  (2) avoiding the use of soaps and other astringents
  (3) removal of the dried secretions that may accumulate on the nipples
  (4) gently massaging a small amount of lanolin into the nipple creases after her bath
  A. All except (2)
  B. (1) and (4)
  C. All of these
  D. (3) and (4)

28. Which of the following is *not* a reason why some doctors may advise against sexual relations during the last month of pregnancy?
  A. to lessen the possibility of abortion
  B. because of the danger of rupturing the membranes
  C. because of the possibility of starting labor prematurely
  D. because of the danger of causing infection

29. Neither Debbie nor Bob smokes; if Debbie did smoke, however, she might be interested to know the effects smoking may have on pregnancy. Smoking seems to be most harmful during the
  A. first 4 months of pregnancy
  B. first 6 months of pregnancy
  C. last 6 months of pregnancy
  D. last 4 months of pregnancy

30. Some studies on the effects of cigarette smoking on pregnancy indicate that
  (1) the more cigarettes smoked by the mother, the lower the infant's birth weight
  (2) the stillbirth rate among smokers is 30% higher than among nonsmokers
  (3) the perinatal mortality rate among smokers is 26% higher than among nonsmokers
  (4) cigarette smoking is even more dangerous when a mother is high risk for other reasons
  A. All of these
  B. (1), (2), and (3)
  C. (2), (3), and (4)
  D. (1) only

31. The nurse needs to establish a relationship of trust with the expectant mother. In order to do this, the nurse needs to
  (1) recognize that first impressions are very important
  (2) be an understanding and intelligent listener as the patient expresses her needs
  (3) do all that she can to make the patient feel accepted and comfortable
  (4) show respect for the mother as an individual
  A. (1) and (4)
  B. (3) and (4)
  C. (2) and (4)
  D. All of these

32. Which of the following would *not* be a way the nurse can show concern for the mother's feelings?
  A. explaining procedures before they are done
  B. avoiding unnecessary exposure of the patient's body during procedures
  C. leaving the room while the doctor examines the mother
  D. providing privacy

33. While assisting the doctor during an examination, the nurse can best help the mother to relax by
  A. telling her to relax
  B. telling her to breathe normally and to keep her back flat against the table
  C. telling her to hold her breath and to lift her back off the table
  D. holding her hand and telling her to lift her back off the table

_C_ **34.** The nurse needs to go over with the mother the instructions the doctor has given her so that the nurse
   (1) can correct any misunderstandings the mother has
   (2) will know what the doctor has told the mother
   (3) can clarify what the doctor was trying to tell the mother
   (4) can find out how the mother intends to carry them out
   A. All of these
   B. All except (1)
   C. All except (2)
   D. All except (4)

_A_ **35.** In counseling the expectant mother regarding nutrition, the nurse is more likely to be successful if she
   (1) first develops a relationship of trust with the mother
   (2) begins her counseling early in pregnancy
   (3) helps the mother to see why changes in her diet are important
   (4) learns the present eating habits of the mother
   A. All of these
   B. All except (1)
   C. All except (2)
   D. All except (4)

_A_ **36.** When helping a mother to utilize her food budget more efficiently, the nurse can suggest that
   (1) dried beans, peas, and peanut butter are inexpensive sources of protein
   (2) fortified skim milk, evaporated milk, and dried milk can be used in place of fresh, whole milk
   (3) breads and cereals made with whole grain or enriched flour provide more nutrients for the same price than those not made with these
   (4) tomatoes are a good source of vitamin C and may be less expensive than citrus fruit at certain times of the year
   A. All of these
   B. (2) and (3)
   C. (1), (2), and (3)
   D. (2), (3), and (4)

_D_ **37.** If Debbie is bothered by constipation during pregnancy, you would advise her *not* to try to correct it by
   A. eating more fresh fruits
   B. eating more raw vegetables
   C. drinking more fluids
   D. leaving milk out of her diet

_C_ **38.** Which of the following suggestions would *not* be appropriate when counseling an expectant mother who is underweight or who has dietary deficiencies?
   A. eat more and larger servings of the basic four food groups
   B. add dried milk to mashed potatoes, meatloafs, cereals
   C. substitute skim milk for whole milk
   D. drink eggnogs or milkshakes and have between-meal snacks

_D_ **39.** Which of the following suggestions would *not* be appropriate when counseling an expectant mother who is overweight?
   A. prepare her food in ways other than frying
   B. decrease the amount of food she eats
   C. increase her activity
   D. eat more and larger servings of the basic four food groups

_B_ **40.** Which of the following potential nursing diagnoses for a pregnant woman is *most* likely to be appropriate for a pregnant teenager?
   A. alteration in comfort related to normal body changes during pregnancy
   B. alteration in nutrition, less than needed for pregnancy and the developing fetus
   C. anxiety related to the condition of the infant
   D. anxiety related to her own health

A **41.** The nurse should try to help the teenage expectant mother see the importance of proper nutrition by helping her to realize that, through an adequate diet
(1) she will have healthier, more attractive skin and hair
(2) her weight will be easier to control
(3) she will have fewer temptations to eat high-calorie foods that are less nourishing
(4) her decisions about food intake will affect the health of her baby
A. All of these
B. (4) only
C. (3) and (4)
D. All except (1)

C **42.** Which of the following would be important data for developing a nursing care plan for an expectant woman?
Information regarding her
(1) financial status
(2) support system
(3) coping mechanisms
(4) feelings toward this pregnancy
(5) health status
A. (5) only
B. (2), (3), and (4)
C. All of these
D. All except (1)

C **43.** Who of the following was not a founder of a method of natural childbirth?
A. Read
B. Bradley
C. Pavlov
D. Lamaze

II. In the space before the procedure in Column I, place the letter or letters from Column II to indicate at which antepartal visit the procedure is usually done.

I PROCEDURE	II ANTEPARTAL VISIT
A **1.** Complete physical examination	**A.** At the first antepartal visit only
A **2.** Obtain medical history	
C **3.** Pelvic examination	**B.** At each antepartal visit
A **4.** Complete urinalysis	
B **5.** Check weight	**C.** Periodically through-out pregnancy
B **6.** Check blood pressure	
B **7.** Test urine for sugar and albumin	**D.** At each visit after the fourth or fifth month
A **8.** Blood test for syphilis	
A **9.** Determine blood type and Rh	**E.** Between the 28th and 32nd week of pregnancy
C **10.** Check hemoglobin and hematocrit	
A **11.** Pap smear	**F.** Last weeks of pregnancy
B **12.** Check for swelling of face or fingers	
B **13.** Question about bleeding	
B **14.** Abdomen palpated, height of uterus measured	
D **15.** Listen to fetal heart tones	
A **16.** Check for immunity against measles, polio etc.	
E **17.** Do roll-over test	
B **18.** Provide opportunity for questions	
F **19.** Instruct regarding signs labor is starting	
B **20.** Question regarding her general well-being	
B **21.** Question about constipation, headaches, indigestion	

III. All of the signs in Column I should be reported to the doctor. Some are danger signs, some are signs labor may be starting. In the space before the sign in Column I, place the letter from Column II which indicates the type of sign it is.

I
SIGN

II
TYPE OF SIGN

_B_ **1.** A trickle or gush of fluid from the vagina

_A_ **2.** Bleeding

_A_ **3.** Rapid weight gain

_B_ **4.** Pink, mucous vaginal discharge (show)

_A_ **5.** Swelling of hands and face

_A_ **6.** Persistent headache

_A_ **7.** Dizziness

_B_ **8.** Intermittent, regular uterine contractions

_A_ **9.** Visual disturbances

_A_ **10.** Persistent vomiting

A. Danger sign

B. Sign labor may be starting

IV. In the space in Column I, place the letter of the discomfort that would be prevented or relieved by the suggestion in Column III. Likewise, in the space in Column II, place the letter of the probable cause of the discomfort in Column I.

I DISCOMFORT	II PROBABLE CAUSE	III SUGGESTIONS FOR PREVENTING OR RELIEVING
1. _F_	1. _a_	**1.** Elastic stockings or bandages to support vessel walls; elevating legs at right angles several times a day
2. _K_	2. _b_	**2.** Relieve constipation
3. _J_	3. _K_	**3.** Increase fluid intake; bathe with soda bicarbonate or take starch or oatmeal bath; use a bland soap or avoid soaps; use oil on skin following bath
4. _C_	4. _d_	**4.** Daily exercise; drink plenty of fluids; eat fruits, vegetables, dark breads, coarse foods; regular time for elimination
5. _E_	5. _c_	**5.** Good body alignment; minimize stooping and lifting; bend at the knees, keeping back straight and feet wide apart; pelvic rocking exercises, abdominal supports; adequate rest
6. _B_	6. _f_	**6.** Avoid fatigue; eat frequent small meals instead of three large ones; reduce fat intake; antacids prescribed by the doctor
7. _L_	7. _e_	**7.** Stretch arms above head while lying flat on back
8. _H_	8. _i_	**8.** Stand up; extend leg with toes pointed toward knee, ankle flexed; heat and massage to leg
9. _D_	9. _g_	**9.** Eat small meals; chew food well; regular elimination; omit gas-forming foods from diet
10. _A_	10. _j_	**10.** Eat dry toast or cracker before getting up in the morning; eat five or six small meals a day instead of three large ones
11. _I_	11. _h_	**11.** Treatment prescribed by the doctor depending on cause, e.g., vinegar douche, suppository, penicillin
12. _G_	12. _l_	**12.** Rest; elevate legs at right angles several times a day

DISCOMFORT	PROBABLE CAUSE
A. Nausea and vomiting	**a.** Standing or sitting for long periods of time; garments that constrict leg vessels
B. Heartburn	**b.** Pressure of uterus on pelvic veins; straining at stool
C. Constipation	**c.** Postural changes during pregnancy; relaxation of sacroiliac joints and symphysis pubis; weak abdominal muscles
D. Flatulence	
E. Backache	**d.** Decreased peristalsis of intestine and decreased tone of abdominal muscles
F. Varicose veins	
G. Swelling of feet	**e.** Crowding of diaphragm by enlarging uterus
H. Leg cramps	**f.** Crowding and decreased motility of stomach with spilling of stomach contents back into esophagus with irritation of lining of esophagus
I. Vaginal infection	
J. Itching	
K. Hemorrhoids	**g.** Relaxation of bowel; undesirable bacterial action
L. Shortness of breath	**h.** *Trichomonas vaginalis, Candida albicans,* gonococcus organism
	i. Seepage of fluid through walls of distended veins
	j. Physiological changes of pregnancy or emotional factors
	k. Dry skin, irritating materials secreted by skin glands, or excessive use of soap
	l. Tension, circulatory impairment caused by pressure of uterus on pelvic veins, overstretching of muscles and fascia of legs; lack of calcium

V. DISCUSSION: Briefly discuss:

1. The effect medication for pain relief may have on the patient's attitude toward herself, her husband, her labor, her child, and future pregnancies

2. How the antepartal care the unmarried pregnant woman typically receives differs from what the married pregnant woman receives, and the effect this has on the pregnancy and its outcome

VI. PROJECTS: Using the telephone directory, community resources directory, or other available sources of information, find out:

1. Which hospitals in your community provide classes for expectant parents, when the classes are held, the number of classes in a series, who teaches them (nurse, doctor, or other person), the cost to the expectant parents, and, briefly, the contents of the classes

Name of hospital:

Day and time classes are held:

Number of classes in a series:

Taught by:

Cost to the expectant parents:

Contents of the classes:

2. Where classes for natural childbirth are held, which method (Lamaze, Bradley etc.) is taught, when the classes are held, how many classes are in a series, who teaches them (nurse, doctor, or other person), the cost to the expectant parents, and, briefly, the contents of the classes

Location:

Method:

Day and time classes are held:

Number of classes in a series:

Taught by:

Cost to the expectant parents:

Contents of the classes:

3. Whether the Red Cross and/or the public health department in your community have classes for expectant parents. If so, when and where they are held, how many are in a series, who teaches them, the cost to the expectant parents, and, briefly, the contents of the classes

	RED CROSS	PUBLIC HEALTH DEPARTMENT

Location:

Day and time classes
are held:

Number of classes in
a series:

Taught by:

Cost to expectant parents:

Contents of the classes:

4. Which facilities in your community provide classes for: siblings; grandparents; couples anticipating cesarean birth

5. Which facilities in your community have birthing rooms; jacuzzis in the labor rooms. Where the nearest alternative birthing center is to your area

I.

1. A	12. D	23. D	34. C
2. C	13. D	24. B	35. A
3. D	14. A	25. A	36. A
4. B	15. C	26. D	37. D
5. A	16. A	27. C	38. C
6. C	17. A	28. A	39. D
7. D	18. C	29. C	40. B
8. B	19. C	30. A	41. A
9. C	20. B	31. D	42. C
10. B	21. A	32. C	43. C
11. A	22. C	33. B	

II.

1. A	7. B	13. B	19. F
2. A	8. A	14. B	20. B
3. C	9. A	15. D	21. B
4. A	10. C	16. A	
5. B	11. A	17. E	
6. B	12. B	18. B	

III.

1. B	4. B	7. A	10. A
2. A	5. A	8. B	
3. A	6. A	9. A	

IV. *Column I*

1. F	7. L
2. K	8. H
3. J	9. D
4. C	10. A
5. E	11. I
6. B	12. G

Column II

1. a	7. e
2. b	8. l
3. k	9. g
4. d	10. j
5. c	11. h
6. f	12. i

assessment of the fetal 9 condition

I. SITUATION: While working in the doctor's office on May 13, you become acquainted with Mrs. R., who is seeing her obstetrician-gynecologist because of irregular menstrual periods. In obtaining her history you find that Mr. and Mrs. R. have been married for 19 years and have 2 adopted children: a daughter who is almost 11 years old and a son who is 6 years old. Mrs. R. is 36 years old, 5'-1" tall. She weighs 260 lb. Four years after their marriage, Mr. and Mrs. R. had an infertility work-up in Montana. The doctors could find no reason for their inability to have children. Four years later they had another work-up at Yale and again the findings were normal. At this time Mrs. R. was given fertility drugs with no result. They decided to adopt. Two years ago Mrs. R. was diagnosed as a mild diabetic and was treated with oral medication.

During his examination on May 13, the doctor diagnosed Mrs. R. as pregnant. She said she thought her last normal menstrual period began December 14. However, because of her obesity and her history of irregular periods, it was difficult for the doctor to determine just how far along the pregnancy was. He discussed with her the effects diabetes can have on pregnancy and recommended that she see her internist at once so that he could evaluate her diabetes. The doctor also suggested doing an amniocentesis for possible fetal abnormalities, but Mrs. R. refused, saying they would not have the pregnancy terminated even if the findings indicated there were abnormalities. The doctor requested that she be seen by him on a weekly basis.

On May 16, Mrs. R. was seen by her internist, who took her off her oral medication for diabetes and put her on 15 units NPH insulin daily. He also requested that Mrs. R. be seen by him every week.

On May 20 and 27, Mrs. R. was seen by her obstetrician and all appeared well. During her visit on June 3, her blood pressure was elevated, so the doctor advised her to limit her activity and to include morning and afternoon rest periods in her daily schedule.

On June 10, the doctor ordered a series of three ultrasound scans for fetal age to be done at weekly intervals.

On June 17, Mrs. R.'s blood pressure was elevated again and the doctor advised that she stay in bed except for going to the bathroom. He also said she could go to the table for meals, although someone else should prepare the meals. He ordered a series of three blood estriols to be done every other day. These were normal.

On June 24, Mrs. R.'s blood pressure was elevated and she had 1+ protein in her urine. The doctor had her admitted to the hospital for treatment. On June 26, Mrs. R. had an oxytocin challenge test (OCT) which was negative. On June 27, she had her third ultrasound scan, which indicated that she was almost 38 weeks pregnant; the fetal weight was estimated as 2,739 g. Since her blood pressure had returned to normal and there was no more protein in her urine, she was discharged from the hospital at 1 P.M. that day. She went home and took a nap. Between 3 and 4 P.M. she was awakened by pain in her lower abdomen. At 8:15 P.M. she was readmitted to the hospital in labor. At 2:52 A.M. on June 28 she gave birth to an 8 lb. 8 oz. (3,856 g) baby girl.

Place the letter of the *best* answer in the space before the statement.

_____ **1.** If you were to classify Mrs. R.'s diabetes according to the age at onset, duration, and vascular involvement, you would say she best fits into class
  A. A
  B. B
  C. C
  D. D

_D_ **2.** Other classifications of diabetes that would apply to Mrs. R. include
   (1) juvenile
   (2) adult
   (3) pregestational
   (4) gestational
   A. (1) and (3)
   B. (1) and (4)
   C. (2) and (4)
   D. (2) and (3)

_A_ **3.** Pregnant diabetics in Mrs. R.'s classification usually
   A. go through pregnancy with few or no complications
   B. have a high maternal mortality rate
   C. have SGA babies
   D. have to have a cesarean section

_C_ **4.** The most likely reason the internist changed Mrs. R.'s treatment from oral medication to insulin is because
   A. insulin is the only medication that can control diabetes effectively
   B. Mrs. R. might have morning sickness and vomit the oral medication
   C. the effect of oral medication on the fetus has not been determined
   D. insulin is less expensive than oral medication

_A_ **5.** If Mrs. R. is correct about her last normal menstrual period, her estimated date of confinement would be
   A. September 21
   B. July 17
   C. August 7
   D. June 7

_B_ **6.** If Mrs. R. is correct about when her last menstrual period began, when she was diagnosed as being pregnant she was already about
   A. 15 weeks pregnant
   B. 25 weeks pregnant
   C. 35 weeks pregnant
   D. 40 weeks pregnant

_D_ **7.** If Mrs. R. had consented to an amniocentesis, you could have explained this procedure to her by saying that it
   A. involves sending high-frequency sound waves into her body and receiving any echoes which then return
   B. is a stress test by which the response of the fetal heart rate to contractions is assessed
   C. is a way to measure the size of the fetal head without using x-rays
   D. is the withdrawal of some of the fluid surrounding the fetus

_C_ **8.** If you had prepared Mrs. R. for an amniocentesis, you would have instructed her to
   (1) drink lots of fluids before the procedure
   (2) refrain from drinking fluids before the procedure
   (3) empty her bladder before the procedure
   (4) be sure her bladder is full before the procedure
   A. (1) and (4)
   B. (2) only
   C. (3) only
   D. (2) and (3)

_A_ **9.** If Mrs. R. had asked you if it hurts when an amniocentesis is done, you should have explained that
   A. the needle prick when the local anesthetic is injected will hurt a little and she may have a sensation of pressure in her pelvis
   B. it is painless
   C. she will be given a general anesthetic so she will feel no pain
   D. the intensity of the contractions may cause some slight discomfort

_A_ **10.** If Mrs. R. had had an amniocentesis, after it was completed you could have instructed her to report to the doctor if she had
(1) vaginal spotting
(2) mild uterine cramps
(3) leakage of fluid
(4) frequency of urination
A. (1) and (3)
B. (2) and (4)
C. (1) and (2)
D. (3) and (4)

_B_ **11.** Amniocentesis is done most often to detect infants with
A. fetal distress
B. Down's syndrome
C. Tay-Sachs disease
D. Duchenne's muscular dystrophy

_D_ **12.** There is usually a sufficient amount of fluid to permit amniocentesis by the
A. 8th or 9th week of pregnancy
B. 10th or 11th week of pregnancy
C. 12th or 13th week of pregnancy
D. 15th or 16th week of pregnancy

_A_ **13.** Meconium in the amniotic fluid is a significant finding during amniocentesis because it indicates a decreased oxygen supply to the fetus. This is true *except* in
A. breech presentations
B. vertex presentations
C. suspected cases of postmaturity
D. suspected cases of intrauterine growth retardation

_A_ **14.** Studies of amniotic fluid that are done to determine fetal maturity include
(1) fat content of squamous cells
(2) creatinine levels
(3) lecithin-sphingomyelin ratio
(4) bilirubin levels
A. All except (4)
B. All of these
C. (3) only
D. (1) and (2)

_C_ **15.** If Mrs. R. had permitted amniocentesis, the doctor may have requested that the lecithin-sphingomyelin (L/S) ratio of the fluid be determined. This ratio is very helpful in assessing the maturity of the fetal
A. neurological system
B. kidneys
C. pulmonary system
D. liver

_A_ **16.** It has been found that the fetal lungs are mature, and therefore respiratory distress syndrome is not likely to occur, when the L/S ratio is at least
A. 2:1
B. 1:8
C. 1:2
D. 1:5

_D_ **17.** The amniotic fluid study that indicates how severely the fetus of an Rh-sensitized mother is being affected by antibodies from the maternal circulation is the determination of the
A. fat content of squamous cells
B. creatinine levels
C. lecithin-sphingomyelin ratio
D. bilirubin levels

_B_ **18.** The blood estriols ordered by the doctor are helpful in determining whether or not the
(1) maternal renal function is normal
(2) placenta is functioning normally
(3) fetal renal function is normal
(4) maternal adrenals are functioning normally
A. (1) only
B. (2) only
C. (1) and (2)
D. (3) and (4)

_B_ **19.** The doctor would know that the fetus was endangered if the estriol levels were
  A. rising
  B. falling
  C. high
  D. remaining the same

_C_ **20.** When explaining the ultrasound scan procedure to Mrs. R., you could say that it
  (1) is a painless procedure
  (2) is a means of measuring the size of the fetal head without x-ray
  (3) is similar to x-ray but does not have the potentially harmful effects of x-ray
  (4) takes about 20 minutes
  A. (1) and (4)
  B. (2) and (3)
  C. All of these
  D. None of these

_D_ **21.** Before the ultrasound is done, you would instruct Mrs. R. to
  (1) avoid eating and drinking
  (2) eat solid foods
  (3) empty her bladder
  (4) be sure her bladder is full
  A. (1) and (3)
  B. (2) and (3)
  C. (3) only
  D. (4) only

_A_ **22.** In addition to determining fetal age, ultrasound can be used to
  (1) locate the placenta
  (2) diagnose multiple pregnancies
  (3) reveal the presence of certain anomalies
  (4) assess maturity of the fetal pulmonary system
  A. All except (4)
  B. (1) and (2)
  C. All except (3)
  D. All of these

_B_ **23.** Ultrasound real-time is useful in
  A. locating the placenta
  B. detecting fetal heartbeat
  C. determining the size of the fetal head
  D. determining the length of labor

_C_ **24.** Mrs. R.'s obstetrician might have ordered x-rays to determine fetal maturity. The fetus is considered to be at term when x-rays show
  (1) characteristic overlapping of the fetal skull bones (Spalding's sign)
  (2) exaggerated curvature of the fetal spine and gas in the fetus
  (3) calcification of the distal femoral epiphyses
  (4) calcification of the proximal tibial epiphyses
  A. (1) and (2)
  B. All of these
  C. (3) and (4)
  D. All except (2)

_B_ **25.** Mrs. R.'s doctor could have ordered x-ray pelvimetry to help in diagnosing
  A. fetal maturity
  B. cephalopelvic disproportion
  C. fetal abnormalities
  D. fetal death

_A_ **26.** The fetal soft tissues could have been evaluated by use of
  A. amniography
  B. amniocentesis
  C. x-ray pelvimetry
  D. blood or urinary estriols

_D_ **27.** The purpose of the oxytocin challenge test (OCT) that Mrs. R. had was to find out if the fetus
  A. was mature
  B. had abnormalities
  C. would be able to tolerate labor
  D. was beginning to suffer from uteroplacental insufficiency (UPI)

_C_ **28.** Supplies and equipment needed to conduct an OCT include
  (1) electronic fetal monitor
  (2) intravenous infusion of oxytocin
  (3) mineral oil
  (4) infusion pump
  A. (1) and (3)
  B. All except (2)
  C. All except (3)
  D. All of these

_D_ **29.** When getting Mrs. R. ready for the OCT, preferably you would position her on her
  (1) right side
  (2) left side
  (3) back with the head of the bed in a semi-Fowler's position
  (4) back with the head of the bed flat
  A. (1) only
  B. (1) or (4)
  C. (2) or (4)
  D. (2) or (3)

_A_ **30.** The indications Mrs. R. had for an OCT included
  (1) diabetes
  (2) suspected postmaturity
  (3) intrauterine growth retardation
  (4) preeclampsia
  A. (1) and (4)
  B. (1) only
  C. (1) and (3)
  D. (1) and (2)

_C_ **31.** Mrs. R.'s doctor would not have ordered an OCT if she had
  A. chronic hypertension
  B. sickle cell disease
  C. placenta previa
  D. cyanotic heart disease

_B_ **32.** In order for the OCT to be of value, there must be a
  (1) good recording of the fetal heart rate and contractions
  (2) contraction pattern of 3 to 4 contractions in 30 minutes for a 60-minute period
  (3) contraction pattern of 3 to 4 contractions in 5 minutes for a 30-minute period
  (4) contraction pattern of 3 to 4 contractions in 10 minutes for a 30-minute period
  A. (1) and (2)
  B. (1) and (4)
  C. (1) and (3)
  D. (1) only

_D_ **33.** Mrs. R.'s OCT was negative. This means that
  A. the frequency of the contractions was less than 3 in 10 min and/or it was impossible to tell if there were late decelerations
  B. there were inconsistent, but definite, late decelerations that did not persist with continued contractions
  C. persistent and consistent late decelerations occurred repeatedly with most contractions
  D. the frequency of contractions was at least 3 in 10 min and no late decelerations occurred

_B_ **34.** After Mrs. R. was in active labor, the electronic fetal monitor was used to monitor the fetal heart rate (FHR) and her contractions. Monitoring the FHR during labor is important because the FHR is the best indicator of the
  A. status of her diabetes
  B. adequacy of fetal oxygenation
  C. status of her preeclampsia
  D. progress of labor

_C_ **35.** Fetal hypoxia
  (1) is normal during labor since there is decreased uterine blood flow during contractions
  (2) if untreated, can result in brain damage or death to the fetus
  (3) could occur as a result of Mrs. R.'s diabetes and preeclampsia
  (4) probably would not occur unless Mrs. R. had an overdose of insulin
  A. All of these
  B. All except (4)
  C. (2) and (3)
  D. (1) and (2)

_A_ **36.** Factors that may affect the fetal heart rate include
  (1) those that interfere with the blood flow to the uterus
  (2) those that interfere with the blood flow to the fetus
  (3) certain drugs the mother receives
  (4) certain conditions of the fetus, such as Rh sensitization and postmaturity
  A. All of these
  B. All except (4)
  C. (2) and (3)
  D. (1) and (2)

_B_ **37.** Which of the following would *not* decrease the blood flow to the uterus?
  A. hypertonic uterine contractions
  B. compression of the umbilical cord
  C. diabetes
  D. maternal hypotension

_D_ **38.** Before you applied the external fetal monitor to Mrs. R., you would
  (1) have her empty her bladder
  (2) be sure her membranes are ruptured and her cervix is 3 to 4 cm dilated
  (3) position her comfortably on her side
  (4) position her comfortably on her back with the bed flat
  A. (3) only
  B. (2) only
  C. (1) and (4)
  D. (1) and (3)

_D_ **39.** Probably the best way to monitor the fetal heart rate during Mrs. R.'s labor is the
  A. fetoscope
  B. Doppler probe
  C. external electronic fetal monitor
  D. internal electronic fetal monitor

_C_ **40.** Which of the following would require intervention if it appeared during Mrs. R.'s labor while the internal fetal monitor was being used?
  (1) loss of baseline variability
  (2) early decelerations
  (3) accelerations
  (4) late decelerations
  A. (1) only
  B. (2) and (3)
  C. (1) and (4)
  D. All of these

_B_ **41.** Which of the following would *not* require intervention if it appeared during Mrs. R.'s labor while the internal fetal monitor was being used?
  (1) baseline variability
  (2) early decelerations
  (3) accelerations
  (4) late decelerations
  A. All of these
  B. All except (4)
  C. (1) and (4)
  D. (2) and (3)

_D_ **42.** Variable decelerations may or may not be a sign of fetal distress. This pattern is *not* considered a sign of fetal distress when
   (1) the heart rate does not stay down to 60 to 70 for more than 30 seconds
   (2) it is not associated with a slow return to baseline
   (3) it is not associated with a rising baseline heart rate
   (4) it is not associated with a loss of variability
   A. (1) and (4)
   B. (2) and (3)
   C. All except (2)
   D. All of these

_A_ **43.** The most common deceleration pattern seen is
   A. variable decelerations
   B. bradycardia
   C. late decelerations
   D. early decelerations

_C_ **44.** The deceleration pattern that is most likely to indicate inadequate fetal oxygenation due to uteroplacental insufficiency is
   A. variable decelerations
   B. bradycardia
   C. late decelerations
   D. early decelerations

_B_ **45.** Variable decelerations are most often caused by
   A. maternal fever
   B. compression of the umbilical cord
   C. uteroplacental insufficiency
   D. compression of the fetal head

_D_ **46.** Early decelerations are most often caused by
   A. maternal fever
   B. compression of the umbilical cord
   C. uteroplacental insufficiency
   D. compression of the fetal head

_A_ **47.** Which of the following is *not* a risk when obtaining blood samples from the fetus in utero?
   A. prolapse of the cord
   B. infection
   C. bleeding
   D. blade breakage

II. A. In the space before the term in Column I, place the letter of its definition from Column II.

I TERM	II DEFINITION
_E_ **1.** Accelerations	**A.** A baseline fetal heart rate (FHR) over 160 beats per minute
_C_ **2.** Baseline	
_F_ **3.** Baseline variability	**B.** A baseline FHR below 120 beats per minute
_B_ **4.** Bradycardia	**C.** FHR recorded between contractions over a period of at least 10 minutes when the internal scalp electrode is in place
_I_ **5.** Decelerations	
_D_ **6.** Early decelerations	**D.** Uniform slowing of the FHR beginning with the onset of the contraction and returning to baseline as the contraction ends
_H_ **7.** Late decelerations	
_A_ **8.** Tachycardia	**E.** Short-term increases in FHR above the baseline
_G_ **9.** Variable deceleration	**F.** Normal beat-to-beat fluctuations of FHR
	G. Nonuniform slowing of FHR which bears no constant time relationship to contractions
	H. Slowing of FHR which begins at, or soon after, the peak of the contraction and does not return to normal until well after the contraction ends
	I. Short-term decreases in FHR below the baseline

B. In the space before the fetal heart rate (FHR) pattern in Column I, place the letter or letters of the intervention indicated from Column II when that pattern appears during electronic fetal monitoring during labor.

	I	II
	FHR PATTERN	INTERVENTION INDICATED

_____   **1.** Accelerations

_____   **2.** Baseline variability

_____   **3.** Bradycardia

_____   **4.** Early decelerations

_____   **5.** Late decelerations that persist

_____   **6.** Loss of baseline variability

_____   **7.** Tachycardia

_____   **8.** Severe variable decelerations

A. Administer O_2

B. Change mother's position, preferably to her left side

C. Decrease uterine activity, if possible

D. Correct maternal hypotension, if present

E. None

F. Prepare for immediate delivery if FHR pattern has not returned to normal within 30 minutes

G. Notify doctor

III. PROJECTS

1. Find out if there are facilities for ultrasound scanning at your hospital. If so, arrange to observe the procedure as it is performed on a pregnant woman.

2. Find out if amniocentesis is done by the obstetricians who practice at your hospital.

   A. If so, is it done most often in the doctor's office or in the hospital?

   B. What studies are done most often on the amniotic fluid?

3. Are electronic fetal monitors used at your hospital?

   A. What type of electronic fetal monitors are used?

   B. Who (MD, RN, LPN) applies the internal scalp electrode and catheter when internal monitoring is done?

C. Who (MD, RN, LPN) is responsible for interpreting the tracings when electronic fetal monitoring is done?

D. What is done with the recordings after the patient has delivered?

E. How are the fetal monitors cleaned after use?

I.

1. B	13. A	25. B	37. B
2. D	14. A	26. A	38. D
3. A	15. C	27. D	39. D
4. C	16. A	28. C	40. C
5. A	17. D	29. D	41. B
6. B	18. B	30. A	42. D
7. D	19. B	31. C	43. A
8. C	20. C	32. B	44. C
9. A	21. D	33. D	45. B
10. A	22. A	34. B	46. D
11. B	23. B	35. C	47. A
12. D	24. C	36. A	

II. A.

1. E	4. B	7. H
2. C	5. I	8. A
3. F	6. D	9. G

B.

1. E	5. A, B, C, D, F, G
2. E	6. A, B, C, D, F, G
3. E	7. A, B, C, D
4. E	8. A, B, C, D, F, G

process of normal 10 labor

I. SITUATION: Debbie and Bob are anticipating the birth of their first baby. They have read all the literature available to them on the birth process, have attended classes for expectant parents, and are receptive to all information you can provide them on the subject.

Place the letter of the *best* answer in the space before the statement.

B 1. When Debbie and Bob ask you what causes labor to start, you tell them it is probably caused by
   (1) an increased production of the hormone oxytocin as pregnancy reaches term
   (2) a decreased production of the hormone oxytocin as pregnancy reaches term
   (3) relaxation of the uterine muscle due to "dropping" of the fetus as pregnancy reaches term
   (4) increased irritability of the uterine muscles due to distension of the muscles as pregnancy reaches term
   A. (1) and (3)
   B. (1) and (4)
   C. (2) and (4)
   D. (2) and (3)

D 2. When Debbie and Bob ask how they will know when labor starts, you tell them that if Debbie experiences any of the following she can expect labor to start soon:
   (1) lightening
   (2) false labor
   (3) heavy bleeding
   (4) spontaneous rupture of the membranes
   A. All of these
   B. (1), (2), and (3)
   C. (2), (3), and (4)
   D. (1), (2), and (4)

A 3. In explaining to Debbie and Bob about lightening, you tell them that
   (1) it is the settling of the fetus into the pelvis
   (2) Debbie will be able to breathe more easily after it happens
   (3) Debbie may have frequency of urination after it happens
   (4) Debbie may experience leg cramps after it happens
   A. All of these
   B. (1), (2), and (3)
   C. (2), (3), and (4)
   D. (1), (2), and (4)

C 4. In discussing false labor with them, you explain that the main difference between false labor and true labor is that
   A. in false labor the contractions are relieved by walking
   B. in false labor the contractions are felt in the abdomen
   C. in true labor the cervix dilates
   D. in true labor the contractions are felt in the lower back and abdomen

_C_   **5.** The pink-tinged vaginal discharge which Debbie may have just before, or soon after, labor starts is called
- **A.** rupturing of the membranes
- **B.** menstruation
- **C.** show
- **D.** mucus plug

_A_   **6.** If Debbie's membranes rupture before labor starts, she should notify the doctor because
- **(1)** of the danger of the umbilical cord prolapsing
- **(2)** the baby may be born very soon
- **(3)** of the possibility of infection developing
- **(4)** she may hemorrhage
- **A.** (1) and (3)
- **B.** (2) and (4)
- **C.** (2) and (3)
- **D.** (1) and (4)

_C_   **7.** In cases of prolapsed cord,
- **(1)** the umbilical cord would descend the birth canal before the baby's head
- **(2)** the baby's oxygen supply might be cut off because of hemorrhage
- **(3)** the baby's oxygen supply might be cut off because of pressure of the head on the cord
- **(4)** the umbilical cord would descend the birth canal after the baby's head
- **A.** All except (1)
- **B.** (4) only
- **C.** (1) and (3)
- **D.** (2) and (4)

_B_   **8.** If you were to discover that the cord had prolapsed, you should
- **A.** administer oxygen to Debbie
- **B.** relieve the pressure on the cord
- **C.** replace the cord to its proper position
- **D.** give Debbie a transfusion

_D_   **9.** In describing labor contractions to Debbie and Bob, you could say that they
- **(1)** are constant and voluntary
- **(2)** are intermittent and involuntary
- **(3)** may be felt first in the low back and then radiate to the abdomen
- **(4)** are always under the complete control of the mother
- **A.** (1) and (3)
- **B.** (1) and (4)
- **C.** (3) and (4)
- **D.** (2) and (3)

_A_   **10.** The period of relaxation between contractions is important so that
- **A.** the fetal oxygen supply can return to normal
- **B.** the maternal oxygen supply can return to normal
- **C.** the mother can rest
- **D.** the mother's blood pressure can return to normal

_C_   **11.** Which of the following descriptions of contractions is *not* charted during labor?
- **A.** intensity
- **B.** duration
- **C.** decrement
- **D.** frequency

_C_   **12.** The frequency of contractions is determined by timing from
- **A.** the end of one to the beginning of the next one
- **B.** the peak of one to the beginning of the next one
- **C.** the beginning of one to the beginning of the next one
- **D.** the beginning of one to its end

_B_   **13.** The changes that occur in the cervix as a result of uterine contractions include
- **(1)** descent
- **(2)** molding
- **(3)** dilatation
- **(4)** effacement
- **A.** (1) and (2)
- **B.** (3) and (4)
- **C.** (2) and (4)
- **D.** All of these

_C_ **14.** The stage of labor in which the placenta is expelled is the
A. first
B. second
C. third
D. fourth

_A_ **15.** The stage of labor in which dilatation occurs is the
A. first
B. second
C. third
D. fourth

_B_ **16.** The stage of labor in which birth of the baby occurs is the
A. first
B. second
C. third
D. fourth

_D_ **17.** In discussing the birth of the baby, you could tell Debbie and Bob that, in order for the baby to be born, the cervix must dilate completely, or
A. 25 cm
B. 20 cm
C. 15 cm
D. 10 cm

_B_ **18.** Debbie and Bob want to know how long Debbie will be in labor. You can tell them that this varies with individuals but that the average length of the first stage of labor for primigravidae is about
A. 8 hours
B. 12 hours
C. 16 hours
D. 24 hours

_A_ **19.** The average length of the second stage of labor for primigravidae is about
A. 1¼ hours
B. 2 hours
C. 3¼ hours
D. 5 hours

_C_ **20.** The average length of the second stage of labor for multigravidae is
A. 7 hours
B. the same as for primigravidae
C. 30 minutes or less
D. 5 to 15 minutes

_B_ **21.** An example of an amnesic drug that Debbie might be given during first stage labor is
A. pentobarbital (Nembutal)
B. scopolamine
C. promethazine (Phenergan)
D. meperidine (Demerol)

_C_ **22.** An example of a tranquilizing drug that Debbie might receive during labor is
A. pentobarbital
B. scopolamine
C. promethazine
D. meperidine

_A_ **23.** Precautions you would take after administering medication for pain relief during labor include
(1) instructing the patient not to get out of bed
(2) putting side rails up on the bed
(3) checking fetal heart tones and mother's respirations
(4) observing progress of labor closely
A. All of these
B. (4) only
C. (2) and (3)
D. (1) only

_C_ **24.** The forces which propel the baby down the birth canal and out through the vaginal opening during second stage labor include
 (1) tissue resistance
 (2) cervical dilatation
 (3) intra-abdominal pressure
 (4) uterine contractions
 A. None of these
 B. All except (2)
 C. (3) and (4)
 D. (2) and (4)

_B_ **25.** You would remind Debbie that the best way for her to shorten the active phase of first stage labor is by
 A. walking during contractions
 B. relaxing during contractions
 C. pushing during contractions
 D. taking medication for pain relief

_C_ **26.** In a vertex presentation in which the occiput is toward the right and back of the mother's pelvis, the position is abbreviated as
 A. L.O.A.
 B. L.O.P.
 C. R.O.P.
 D. R.O.A.

_B_ **27.** An episiotomy that is made slightly laterally toward the mother's left is abbreviated as
 A. M.L.
 B. L.M.L.
 C. L.S.A.
 D. R.M.L.

_C_ **28.** A laceration in which the mucous membrane, skin, and muscles of the perineum as well as the anal sphincter are involved is called a
 A. first degree
 B. second degree
 C. third degree
 D. fifth degree

_A_ **29.** This type of anesthesia when administered to the mother is probably *least* likely to affect the baby
 A. pudendal block
 B. saddle block
 C. caudal
 D. general

_B_ **30.** Labor is rarely regarded with indifference by the expectant mother. You would expect Debbie to anticipate labor
 A. as a terrifying ordeal
 B. calmly without unnecessary fears
 C. with apprehension because of her inexperience in childbirth
 D. as a test of her endurance

II. In the space before the term in Column I, place the letter of its definition from Column II.

	I TERM		II DEFINITION
I	1. Amniotomy	**A.**	That part of the fetus lowest in the mother's pelvis
C	2. Breech presentation	**B.**	The baby's head is the lowest part in the mother's pelvis
E	3. Engaged	**C.**	The buttocks and/or the feet of the baby are lowest in the mother's pelvis
K	4. Episiotomy		
F	5. Floating	**D.**	The relation of the presenting part to the ischial spines of the mother's pelvis
L	6. Lacerations	**E.**	The widest diameter of the baby's head is at midpelvis
J	7. Molding		
G	8. Position	**F.**	The widest diameter of the baby's head is above midpelvis
A	9. Presentation		
D	10. Station	**G.**	The relation of a certain point on the presenting part to the mother's pelvis
B	11. Vertex presentation		
H	12. Occiput	**H.**	The certain point on the presenting part in a vertex presentation
		I.	Artificial rupture of the membranes by the doctor
		J.	Overlapping of the bones of the baby's head to permit it to fit the birth canal
		K.	An incision into the perineum at the lower border of the vagina to facilitate birth
		L.	Tears

III. From the list below select the correct type of anesthetic to complete the statements. Some answers may be used more than once.

Caudal
General (inhalation)
Local
Pudendal block
Saddle block
Paracervical block
Continuous caudal
Epidural

1. In _General_ anesthesia, the mother is asleep during delivery.

2. When a _pudendal block_ is given, the pudendal nerves supplying the perineum are injected with the anesthetizing drug.

3. In _saddle block_, the anesthetizing drug is injected under the dura of the spinal cord; in _epidural_ it is injected above the dura.

4. When _continuous caudal_ and _epidural_ anesthesia are used, a polyethylene tubing may be inserted and left in place so that additional medication can be injected as needed.

5. When _general_ anesthesia is used, the mother should receive a drying agent first and all personnel and equipment in the delivery room should be conductive.

6. When _local_ anesthesia is used, the drug is injected into the tissues of the perineum where the episiotomy is to be made.

7. _Caudal_ and _epidural_ anesthesia may be started as soon as labor is well established and continued throughout labor and delivery.

8. _Pudendal block_ anesthesia produces marked relaxation of the perineum and thus hastens birth by reducing tissue resistance.

9. _Saddle block_, _caudal_, _pudendal block_, and _epidural_ are examples of regional anesthesia.

10. When _general_ anesthesia is anticipated, the mother is not given foods or fluids in order to lessen the chance of aspiration of vomitus by the mother.

11. _Saddle block_ , _caudal_ , or _epidural_ anesthesia does not affect the baby unless there is a drop in the mother's blood pressure.

12. Prolonged use of _general_ anesthesia before the baby is born may damage the baby.

13. In _paracervical block_ the anesthetic is injected on either side of the cervix.

I.
1. B
2. D
3. A
4. C
5. C
6. A
7. C
8. B
9. D
10. A
11. C
12. C
13. B
14. C
15. A
16. B
17. D
18. B
19. A
20. C
21. B
22. C
23. A
24. C
25. B
26. C
27. B
28. C
29. A
30. B

II.
1. I
2. C
3. E
4. K
5. F
6. L
7. J
8. G
9. A
10. D
11. B
12. H

III.
1. General (inhalation)
2. Pudendal block
3. Saddle block; epidural
4. Continuous caudal, epidural
5. General (inhalation)
6. Local
7. Caudal, epidural
8. Pudendal block
9. Saddle block, caudal, pudendal block, epidural
10. General (inhalation)
11. Saddle block, caudal, epidural
12. General (inhalation)
13. Paracervical block

nursing care during 11 labor

I. **SITUATION:** Debbie and Bob are expecting their first baby. Debbie began her maternity leave from her job 1 month before her estimated date of confinement. She and Bob spent the next 3 weeks completing the nursery and the preparations for the baby. The last week Debbie spent cleaning house and preparing meals that could be frozen for future use.

Bob and Debbie have many friends but no family in the town where they live. After the baby is born they plan to call her mother and she will fly out and spend the next 2 weeks with them. Until she arrives, Bob will do his own cooking or will eat out.

Now, a week past her estimated date of confinement, Debbie's suitcase is packed and everything is ready, but the baby seems content to stay in its cozy surroundings. In order to help pass the time, Debbie agreed to go shopping with a friend this afternoon. Around 2:30 P.M. she felt a cramp in her low abdomen; about 20 minutes later she felt another cramp. Since they only lasted a few seconds she passed them off as insignificant, although she did note the frequency with which they were occurring. By the time she arrived home at 5 P.M., her "cramps" were regular contractions coming at 5-minute intervals and lasting 30 to 40 seconds. She had Bob's dinner ready for him when he arrived home at 6 P.M. She did not eat. Debbie's contractions were coming at 4-minute intervals and lasting 40 to 50 seconds by the time they arrived at the hospital at 7 P.M.

Debbie and Bob plan to have natural childbirth.

Place the letter of the *best* answer in the space before the statement.

_C_ 1. When admitting Debbie, you can help to make her feel comfortable and at ease by
   (1) greeting her warmly
   (2) introducing yourself
   (3) hurriedly completing the admission procedures
   (4) using technical medical terms when explaining procedures
   A. All of these
   B. All except (3)
   C. (1) and (2)
   D. (1) and (4)

_C_ 2. Your assessments of Debbie on admission would include
   (1) the time her labor started
   (2) the status of her membranes
   (3) her support system
   (4) effacement, dilatation, station, and presentation
   (5) fetal heart rate and vital signs
   A. (1), (4), and (5)
   B. (1), (3), and (5)
   C. All of these
   D. All except (3)

_B_ 3. You would consider that Debbie's labor started at
   A. 2:30 P.M.
   B. 5 P.M.
   C. 6 P.M.
   D. 7 P.M.

_D_ **4.** Which of the following laboratory tests probably would *not* be ordered for Debbie as part of the admission procedure?
 (1) urinalysis
 (2) blood group and Rh
 (3) CBC
 (4) type and cross-match two units of blood
 A. (1) and (2)
 B. (2) and (3)
 C. (1) and (4)
 D. (2) and (4)

_A_ **5.** The purpose of the vaginal exam of Debbie on admission was to obtain information regarding the
 (1) presentation and postion of the baby
 (2) effacement and dilatation of the cervix
 (3) station of the presenting part
 (4) presence and amount of bloody show
 A. All except (4)
 B. All except (1)
 C. (2) only
 D. (1) and (3)

_C_ **6.** Your preparation of Debbie for labor and delivery probably will include
 (1) a shave
 (2) an amniotomy
 (3) an episiotomy
 (4) an enema
 A. All of these
 B. (1) only
 C. (1) and (4)
 D. (2) and (3)

_D_ **7.** If Debbie were in advanced labor on admission, which of the preparatory procedures would you probably omit?
 A. shave
 B. amniotomy
 C. episiotomy
 D. enema

_B_ **8.** Debbie says she has never had an enema and asks why she has to have one now. You explain that an enema is given to
 (1) allow the doctor to see where to do the episiotomy
 (2) make more room for the baby as it descends the birth canal
 (3) prevent her from having a bowel movement during the birth
 (4) stimulate labor
 A. All of these
 B. All except (1)
 C. (2) and (3)
 D. All except (4)

_A_ **9.** You observe the progress of Debbie's labor by
 (1) timing her contractions
 (2) noting her reaction to her contractions
 (3) noting the presence and amount of bloody show
 (4) examining her
 A. All of these
 B. (1) and (4)
 C. All except (2)
 D. (2) and (3)

_C_ **10.** When taking Debbie's vital signs on admission you would
 (1) take her blood pressure between contractions
 (2) take her blood pressure during contractions
 (3) report a blood pressure of 140/90 or higher to the doctor
 (4) report a blood pressure of less than 120/80 to the doctor
 A. (1) and (4)
 B. (2) and (4)
 C. (1) and (3)
 D. (2) and (3)

_D_ **11.** The goal of emotional support for Debbie during labor is to
   (1) help her cope in a satisfying manner during labor and the birth
   (2) help enhance her self-image
   (3) help her develop positive attitudes toward Bob and their child
   (4) help her develop positive attitudes toward future pregnancies
   A. (1) only
   B. (2) and (3)
   C. (1) and (4)
   D. All of these

_A_ **12.** Bob can provide emotional support for Debbie during labor by
   (1) staying with her
   (2) entertaining her
   (3) coaching her in relaxation and breathing techniques
   (4) praising and encouraging her
   A. All of these
   B. All except (2)
   C. (4) only
   D. (1) and (4)

_D_ **13.** Labor patients who would need the most emotional support by the nurse would probably be those who
   (1) have consistently practiced relaxation and breathing techniques
   (2) have obtained information about childbirth from reading
   (3) are laboring alone
   (4) have had an unhappy experience with a previous labor
   A. All of these
   B. (2) and (3)
   C. (2) and (4)
   D. (3) and (4)

_C_ **14.** Some couples who attend childbirth education classes may not perform well during labor because
   (1) they have not practiced their exercises and relaxation techniques
   (2) they have misconceptions about labor
   (3) the husband is not an effective coach
   (4) they are not committed to the method taught
   A. (1) only
   B. All except (2)
   C. All of these
   D. (3) and (4)

_B_ **15.** During the active phase of labor, if the husband is coaching his wife effectively and she is responding well to his coaching, the nurse should
   A. help the husband coach his wife
   B. remain in the room but not interfere
   C. remain at the nurses' station until they call her
   D. remain at the nurses' station but occasionally examine the patient

_A_ **16.** Ways that you can provide emotional support to Debbie during labor might include
   (1) explaining to her and Bob what is happening as labor progresses
   (2) providing a quiet, private atmosphere so that she can concentrate on her breathing and relaxation techniques with as few interruptions as possible
   (3) coaching her while Bob gets something to eat
   (4) being firm if she loses control during contractions
   A. All of these
   B. (1) and (2)
   C. (2) and (4)
   D. (2) and (3)

_C_ **17.** You commend Debbie for not eating after her labor started. Food and fluids may be withheld during labor because
   A. she does not need them during labor
   B. she will be fed intravenously during labor
   C. when labor starts, digestion stops
   D. she may vomit when given general anesthesia for delivery

_D_ **18.** The time when medication for pain relief is given can affect the progress of labor. To be of the most benefit to Debbie without slowing or stopping her labor, the medication probably should be given
  A. whenever Debbie wants it
  B. when her cervix is 8 to 9 cm dilated
  C. when her cervix is 2 to 3 cm dilated
  D. when her cervix is 4 to 5 cm dilated

_A_ **19.** The reason Debbie's bladder should not be allowed to become distended during labor is because a full bladder
  (1) can be injured by labor
  (2) is uncomfortable
  (3) can interfere with uterine contractions
  (4) can prevent descent of the baby
  A. All of these
  B. (1) and (4)
  C. (2) only
  D. (1), (3), and (4)

_C_ **20.** One of the best ways of preventing infection in mother and infant is
  A. separating mothers with infections from other mothers
  B. providing individual equipment for each mother and thoroughly cleansing and sterilizing it before it is used by another patient
  C. frequent and thorough handwashing by all personnel caring for them
  D. preventing anyone with infection from caring for them

_A_ **21.** The *first* thing you would do after Debbie's membranes rupture is
  A. listen to the fetal heart tones
  B. examine her to see how much the cervix is dilated
  C. place a dry pad under her
  D. chart the color and amount of the fluid

_B_ **22.** After her membranes rupture, you would explain to Debbie that
  (1) her contractions will now be milder and more comfortable
  (2) she will continue to lose fluid until the baby is born
  (3) her contractions probably will become stronger and more efficient
  (4) she has no control over the fluid drainage
  A. (1) only
  B. All except (1)
  C. All except (3)
  D. (4) only

_D_ **23.** Which of the following would *not* be considered a sign of fetal distress?
  A. persistent tachycardia
  B. severe variable decelerations or late decelerations that persist
  C. fetal heart rate that slows below 100 beats per minute during contractions and does not return to normal within 10 to 15 seconds after the contraction ends
  D. meconium in the amniotic fluid in a breech presentation

_B_ **24.** Which of the following would *not* be considered a sign of transition?
  A. suddenly the mother is unable to relax during her contractions
  B. the cervix is 4 to 5 cm dilated
  C. the mother becomes nauseated and vomits
  D. the mother gets the "shakes"

_A_ **25.** If, during a contraction, Debbie strains as though trying to have a bowel movement and at the same time makes a deep, grunting sound, you would
  A. suspect that the second stage of labor has begun
  B. suspect that she is in transition
  C. offer her the bedpan
  D. ask her if she would like some medication for pain

_D_ **26.** The best position for Debbie for pushing is
  A. on her left side
  B. on her back with her head elevated
  C. squatting
  D. the one that is most effective

_C_ **27.** Which of the following would you *not* do during second stage labor?
  A. wipe Debbie's face with a cold, damp cloth between pushes
  B. stay with Debbie while she is pushing
  C. encourage Debbie to push between each contraction
  D. explain to Debbie that she will feel more and more pressure as she pushes

_D_ **28.** You would determine the progress of labor while Debbie is pushing by
- **A.** examining her
- **B.** asking her if she can feel the baby lower
- **C.** feeling her abdomen to see if the baby is lower
- **D.** watching her perineum for bulging

Debbie was completely dilated at 12:15 A.M. At 1 A.M. she was taken to the delivery room. Bob changed into a scrub suit and put on a cap, mask, and shoe covers. Then, after washing his hands, he joined Debbie in the delivery room. A stool was provided for him so that he could sit at Debbie's head and coach her. The mirror was adjusted so that he and Debbie could watch the birth. The nurse placed Debbie's legs in stirrups and the short end of the delivery table was recessed under the long end. The nurse then used a Betadine solution and gauze sponges to cleanse Debbie's lower abdomen, thighs, and vulva. Debbie continued to push with each contraction. After putting on a sterile gown and gloves, the doctor placed sterile drapes under Debbie's buttocks and over her legs and abdomen. Bob and Debbie were requested not to touch the top of the drapes. The doctor injected a 1% solution of mepivacaine (Carbocaine) into the area of the pudendal nerves. After the area was numb, the doctor made an incision from the lower border of the vagina down the middle of the perineum. With the next contraction, as Debbie pushed gently according to the doctor's instructions, the baby's head was born. The back of the head appeared first and was toward Debbie's front. As the head was born it rotated so that the back of the head (the occiput) was toward Debbie's left. As soon as the head was born, the doctor slipped a finger along the baby's neck toward its shoulder to see if the cord was around its neck. It was not. He then suctioned the baby's nose and mouth with a rubber bulb syringe. Then the rest of the baby was gently lifted out. The time was 1:20 A.M. A squeal of delight came from both Bob and Debbie as they saw their daughter, Jennifer, enter the world. The baby cried lustily as soon as she was born, then she stopped crying and looked around. Bob had his camera and as soon as the doctor placed her on Debbie's abdomen he began to take pictures. The doctor clamped and cut her cord and then placed her in a heated crib where a warm, sterile receiving blanket was open ready for her. The nurse quickly but gently and thoroughly dried her with the blanket and then placed her on the scale which was covered with a soft towel. She weighed 8 lb 1 oz (3,657 g). The nurse then placed her in the heated crib and wrapped her in another warm receiving blanket. Bob was busy taking pictures and describing her to Debbie while the doctor repaired the episiotomy. At 1:26 A.M. the placenta was delivered and the doctor ordered Syntocinon 10 units I.M. for Debbie. The nurse took Debbie's blood pressure and gave her the Syntocinon.

The nurse wrapped Jennifer snugly in a second blanket and handed her to Bob. He held her close to Debbie and together they inspected her. As soon as the doctor was finished, the drapes were removed, Debbie's vulva was gently cleansed and dried, perineal pads were applied, the short end of the delivery table was replaced, and Debbie's legs were lifted from the stirrups. She was covered with a warm bath blanket and then Jennifer was placed in her arms. Since she planned to breast-feed Jennifer, the nurse helped her onto her side and took her arm out of her gown while Bob held the baby. An extra pillow was placed under her head and the nurse helped her get all the nipple and as much as possible of the areola into Jennifer's mouth. And wonder of wonders, Jennifer nursed! Bob stayed close by to assist if needed. After Jennifer had nursed, Debbie put her gown back on and the nurse took a picture of the three of them.

While Jennifer was nursing, the nurse made the identification bracelets and completed the chart. After Debbie was ready for her to do so, the nurse took Jennifer and instilled the eye medication, applied the bracelets to mother and baby, and footprinted the baby and thumbprinted the mother. Debbie and Bob had brought their baby book so the nurse put Jennifer's footprints in it, too. Then Jennifer and the records pertaining to her were taken to the nursery. Debbie's blood pressure and pulse were taken and the height and tone of her uterus were checked. Her blood pressure was 110/70, pulse 80, and her uterus was firm and even with her umbilicus. She was then taken to the recovery room. Debbie and Bob were happy but tired. They decided Bob should go home and Debbie should rest.

_B_ **29.** The length of the first stage of labor for Debbie was
- **A.** longer than the average for primigravidae
- **B.** shorter than the average for primigravidae
- **C.** shorter than the average for multigravidae
- **D.** the same as the average for primigravidae

_B_ **30.** The type of anesthesia Debbie received was
- **A.** general
- **B.** pudendal block
- **C.** caudal
- **D.** saddle block

_D_ 31. The type of episitomy Debbie had was
A. R.M.L.
B. L.M.L.
C. R.S.L.
D. M.L.

_C_ 32. The position of the baby was
A. R.O.P.
B. L.O.P.
C. L.O.A.
D. R.O.A.

_A_ 33. The purpose of suctioning the baby's mouth and nose is to
A. clear the airway
B. stimulate the baby to cry
C. obtain specimen for culture
D. prevent hemorrhage

_C_ 34. The purpose of clamping the umbilical cord is to
A. prevent infection
B. stimulate the baby to cry
C. prevent hemorrhage
D. prevent cold stress

_D_ 35. The purpose of placing Jennifer in a heated crib and drying her thoroughly is to
A. prevent infection
B. stimulate her to cry
C. prevent hemorrhage
D. prevent cold stress

_B_ 36. The Syntocinon Debbie received after the placenta was delivered is
A. an analgesic
B. an oxytocic
C. a narcotic
D. a hypnotic

_B_ 37. The purpose of the Syntocinon is to
A. relieve Debbie's pain so the doctor can repair her episiotomy
B. prevent Debbie from hemorrhaging by stimulating her uterus to contract
C. relax Debbie so that she can nurse her baby
D. put Debbie to sleep since she has been awake all night

_A_ 38. In order to lessen the danger of hemorrhage, you would prefer Debbie's uterus to be
A. firm and at or below the umbilicus
B. soft and at or below the umbilicus
C. firm and above the umbilicus
D. soft and above the umbilicus

_B_ 39. The main reasons Debbie and Bob were encouraged to hold Jennifer soon after she was born are
(1) to promote parent-infant bonding
(2) so that they could get acquainted with her
(3) so that the nurse could be free to do the paperwork
(4) because breast-feeding causes the uterus to contract and helps prevent postpartum bleeding
(5) so that the nurse wouldn't have to answer their questions about whether she is normal
A. (3) and (5)
B. (1) and (2)
C. (2) and (3)
D. (4) and (5)

_D_ 40. Of the following behavior which you might observe by parents in the delivery room soon after the birth of their baby, which might be signs of rejection of the baby?
(1) holding the baby in the *en face* position
(2) avoiding eye contact with the baby
(3) touching the infant's arms, hands, and face
(4) making statements such as "It sure is ugly! It looks like a wet frog!"
(5) refusing to look at or hold the infant
A. (5) only
B. (1) and (3)
C. (1), (2), and (3)
D. (2), (4), and (5)

II. In Column I are listed some of the physical discomforts that may annoy Debbie during labor. In Column II, opposite the discomfort in Column I, suggest ways the nurse can prevent or relieve the discomfort.

I DISCOMFORTS DURING LABOR	II NURSING INTERVENTIONS TO PREVENT OR RELIEVE
A. Dry, cracked lips	**A.**
B. Dry mouth	**B.**
C. Wetness from amniotic fluid	**C.**
D. Bloody, sticky vulva from show	**D.**
E. Chilly feeling, cold feet	**E.**
F. Hot feeling, perspiring	**F.**

III. PROJECTS

1. Find out what is done with the patient's clothing when she is admitted to the labor suite at your hospital. If it is not sent home, what measures are taken to prevent it from getting lost?

    A. Clothing sent home.

    B. Care of clothing kept at hospital.

2. Find out what types of shaves are done on labor patients at your hospital.

    A. Complete   **B.** Partial (half)   **C.** Partial (episiotomy area only)

3. Find out what regulations your hospital has regarding visitors in the labor suite.

    A. Husbands only

    B. Father of the baby

    C. Childbirth education coaches

    D. Others

4. Find out who is permitted to be with the mother during delivery.

I.
1. C	**11.** D	**21.** A	**31.** D
2. C	**12.** A	**22.** B	**32.** C
3. B	**13.** D	**23.** D	**33.** A
4. D	**14.** C	**24.** B	**34.** C
5. A	**15.** B	**25.** A	**35.** D
6. C	**16.** A	**26.** D	**36.** B
7. D	**17.** C	**27.** C	**37.** B
8. B	**18.** D	**28.** D	**38.** A
9. A	**19.** A	**29.** B	**39.** B
10. C	**20.** C	**30.** B	**40.** D

II.   **A.** Apply petroleum jelly or A & D ointment
   B. Ice chips, if permitted; rinse with mouthwash
   C. Bathe, dry, change underpad
   D. Bathe area, dry
   E. Increase room temperaure; apply blankets, hot water bottle
   F. Lower room temperature; remove blankets; use cold, damp cloth

normal body changes 12 during the puerperium

I. SITUATION: In caring for Debbie the day following the birth of her daughter, Jennifer, you find her full of questions about when she will get back her figure, when her milk will come in, if the bloody discharge is menstruation and how long she'll have it, what causes her to have cramps now, when her episiotomy will be healed, and whether the doctor will have to take out the stitches. While giving her a bath you try to answer her questions and explain the changes she can expect following birth.

Place the letter of the *best* answer in the space before the statement.

B 1. Since Debbie plans to nurse Jennifer, you can explain that the changes that occur in her breasts during the puerperium are due to the lactogenic hormone
  A. chorionic gonadotropin
  B. prolactin
  C. estrogen
  D. progesterone

A 2. As a result of an increased blood supply and an increased glandular activity, Debbie can expect that in about 3 days her breasts will become
  (1) engorged
  (2) hard and painful
  (3) soft and comfortable
  (4) flabby
  A. (1) and (2)
  B. (1) and (3)
  C. (2) and (3)
  D. (2) and (4)

D 3. The first substance Debbie's breasts will secrete is called
  A. milk
  B. lochia
  C. prolactin
  D. colostrum

C 4. Debbie can anticipate that her milk will be in in about
  A. 5 or 6 days
  B. 4 or 5 days
  C. 3 or 4 days
  D. 1 or 2 days

C 5. After lactation is established, Debbie can expect that her breasts will be
  A. engorged
  B. hard and painful
  C. soft and comfortable
  D. flabby

B 6. The processes involved in lactation include the
  (1) secretion of milk
  (2) assimilation of milk
  (3) absorption of milk
  (4) expulsion of milk
  A. (1) and (3)
  B. (1) and (4)
  C. (2) and (3)
  D. (2) and (4)

_D_ **7.** Debbie should know that the lactation process that is controlled by the let-down reflex can be affected by her emotions. This process is the
  A. secretion of milk
  B. assimilation of milk
  C. absorption of milk
  D. expulsion of milk

_A_ **8.** In order for Debbie to get her figure back, the uterus must return to its normal size and position. This process is called
  A. involution
  B. convolution
  C. diuresis
  D. diaphoresis

_C_ **9.** You can tell Debbie that the length of time it takes the uterus to return to its normal size and position is about
  A. 2 weeks
  B. 4 weeks
  C. 6 weeks
  D. 8 weeks

_D_ **10.** In order for the uterus to return to its normal size, certain changes occur in it following delivery. These include
  (1) replacement of the large blood vessels at the placental site with new, smaller ones
  (2) decrease in size of muscle cells in the uterus
  (3) sloughing off and discharge of the outer layer of the decidua
  (4) breaking down and casting out of some of the protein material in the uterine wall
  A. (1) and (3)
  B. (2) and (4)
  C. All except (1)
  D. All of these

_B_ **11.** Although Debbie's uterus can be easily felt in the abdomen for a while after delivery, it probably will have resumed its position as a pelvic organ in about
  A. 5 days
  B. 10 days
  C. 15 days
  D. 20 days

_D_ **12.** In response to Debbie's question about her vaginal discharge, you can tell her it is called
  A. menstruation
  B. diaphoresis
  C. diuresis
  D. lochia

_A_ **13.** Debbie can be told that the vaginal discharge comes from the placental site and indicates the healing that is occurring there. She can expect that she will probably have some discharge for about
  A. 3 weeks
  B. 1 week
  C. 4 weeks
  D. 2 weeks

_B_ **14.** Compared to Mrs. B., who has had four children, you would expect Debbie to have
  A. slightly more lochia
  B. less lochia
  C. the same amount of lochia
  D. considerably more lochia

_C_ **15.** You would suspect Debbie had an infection if her lochia had a
  A. bitter odor
  B. characteristic odor
  C. foul odor
  D. sweet odor

_A_ **16.** Another name for the cramps Debbie experiences during the puerperium is
  A. afterpains
  B. labor pains
  C. diaphoresis
  D. diuresis

_D_ **17.** Afterpains are caused by the
   A. relaxation of the uterus following a period of contraction
   B. relaxation of the uterus before a period of contraction
   C. contraction and retraction of the uterus
   D. contraction of the uterus following a brief period of relaxation

_B_ **18.** Afterpains are more likely to be experienced by a
   A. primipara who breast-feeds
   B. multipara who breast-feeds
   C. primipara who bottle-feeds
   D. multipara who bottle-feeds

_C_ **19.** Although Debbie will not be aware of them, certain changes occur in her cervix following birth. These include
   (1) an increase in the number of muscle cells
   (2) a decrease in the number of muscle cells
   (3) return of the external os to its normal size while the internal os remains slightly dilated
   (4) return of the internal os to its normal size while the external os remains slightly dilated
   A. (1) and (3)
   B. (2) and (4)
   C. (1) and (4)
   D. (2) and (3)

_A_ **20.** Debbie can expect to have her first menstrual period about
   A. 2 months after lactation ceases
   B. 2 months before lactation ceases
   C. 6 weeks after delivery
   D. 8 weeks after delivery

_D_ **21.** When Debbie asks you about the "ugly stretch marks" on her abdomen, you can tell her that usually they become
   A. silvery in appearance then disappear completely
   B. redder in appearance then disappear completely
   C. redder in appearance but do not disappear completely
   D. silvery in appearance but do not disappear completely

_D_ **22.** Debbie is disappointed that she has not lost as much weight as she thought she would when the baby was born. You can explain that she will probably lose another 4 to 5 lb during the next couple of weeks due to
   (1) exercise
   (2) lack of food intake
   (3) diuresis
   (4) diaphoresis
   A. (1) and (2)
   B. (1) and (3)
   C. (2) and (4)
   D. (3) and (4)

_B_ **23.** If Debbie has difficulty urinating, you can explain that this
   (1) is because the urethra is swollen and she is sore
   (2) is temporary and in 24 to 48 hours she will be able to urinate without difficulty
   (3) happens when unusually large babies are born
   (4) happens when unusually large episiotomies are necessary
   A. All of these
   B. (1) and (2)
   C. (3) and (4)
   D. (4) only

_A_ **24.** If Debbie is bothered by constipation following delivery, you can tell her that
   (1) it is due to relaxation of the abdominal wall and loss of intra-abdominal pressure
   (2) the doctor has a laxative and/or enema ordered if she needs it
   (3) this problem will persist now that she has started her family
   (4) this problem is due to her unwillingness to have a bowel movement for fear of breaking her stitches
   A. (1) and (2)
   B. (3) only
   C. (4) only
   D. (2) and (3)

_D_ **25.** After the excitement of the birth and sharing the news about the birth has subsided, Debbie may experience a let-down feeling. This is known as
  A. postpartum exhilaration and occurs about the third day
  B. antepartum exhilaration and occurs about the tenth day
  C. antepartum blues and occurs about the tenth day
  D. postpartum blues and occurs about the third day

_C_ **26.** After the birth of a baby, a couple may have less sexual satisfaction for a while because
  (1) they have less privacy
  (2) their attention is concentrated on the baby instead of on each other
  (3) the wife has less desire for sexual activity
  (4) the husband may be afraid of hurting his wife
  (5) they may be too exhausted
  A. (2), (3), and (4)
  B. (1) only
  C. All of these
  D. All except (5)

II. In the space before the description of the lochia in Column I, place the letter of the lochia it describes from Column II.

	I	II
	DESCRIPTION	LOCHIA
_B_	**1.** Appears third to eighth day	**A.** Lochia rubra
_A_	**2.** Appears first to third day	**B.** Lochia serosa
_C_	**3.** Appears ninth to tenth day	**C.** Lochia alba
_A_	**4.** Red and bloody	
_C_	**5.** Yellowish-white	
_B_	**6.** Serous, pink or brown	

III. PROJECTS

1. By interviewing three obstetricians who are not partners, or by reading the postpartum instructions they give to their patients, find out:

  A. How soon after the mother is discharged from the hospital she is routinely seen by the doctor

  B. What, specifically, the doctor looks for during his postpartum examination

2. Find out what material is used for suture in repairing episiotomies. Does it dissolve or must the doctor remove it after the wound is healed?

I.
1. B
2. A
3. D
4. C
5. C
6. B
7. D

8. A
9. C
10. D
11. B
12. D
13. A
14. B

15. C
16. A
17. D
18. B
19. C
20. A
21. D

22. D
23. B
24. A
25. D
26. C

II.
1. B
2. A
3. C

4. A
5. C
6. B

nursing care during the 13 puerperium

I. **SITUATION:** After Jennifer was born, Debbie and Bob spent several minutes holding her and getting acquainted with her. Then she was taken to the nursery and Debbie was taken to the recovery room. Since Debbie and Bob were tired by then, they decided Bob should go home and Debbie should get some rest.

Place the letter of the *best* answer in the space before the statement.

_C_ 1. In the recovery room Debbie began to shake uncontrollably. This is probably due to
  (1) nervousness and exhaustion
  (2) the cold temperature of the room
  (3) the sudden weight loss
  (4) rapid cooling of the body
  A. All of these
  B. All except (1)
  C. All except (2)
  D. (1) and (2)

_A_ 2. You can best help Debbie overcome the shaky feeling by
  A. keeping her warm
  B. giving her a bath
  C. giving her intravenous fluids
  D. giving her a sedative

_D_ 3. You can give Debbie something to drink if
  A. the doctor orders it
  B. her bladder is not full
  C. her blood pressure is not elevated
  D. she is not nauseated

_B_ 4. Probably the most critical period for Debbie following delivery is the
  A. first 6 hours
  B. first hour
  C. first week
  D. first 24 hours

_A_ 5. While she is in the recovery room, you will check Debbie's
  (1) blood pressure and pulse
  (2) fundus
  (3) lochia
  (4) perineum
  A. All of these
  B. (1) only
  C. (2) and (3)
  D. (2) and (4)

_A_ 6. If you should find Debbie's uterus three fingers above the umbilicus and displaced to one side, you would suspect that
  A. her bladder is full
  B. she is hemorrhaging
  C. this is the normal location at this time
  D. she has a hematoma

_C_   **7.** Following delivery, you want Debbie's uterus to stay contracted. A contracted uterus
- **(1)** is necessary to prevent hemorrhage
- **(2)** feels soft and boggy to the touch
- **(3)** feels firm to the touch
- **(4)** must be massaged
- **A.** (1) and (4)
- **B.** (2) and (3)
- **C.** (1) and (3)
- **D.** (2) and (4)

_D_   **8.** While Debbie is in the recovery room you would expect the amount of her lochia to be
- **A.** scant
- **B.** heavy
- **C.** heavy with clots
- **D.** moderate

_B_   **9.** If Debbie complained of excruciating pain in her stitches or rectum, you would suspect that she has
- **A.** a low pain tolerance
- **B.** a hematoma
- **C.** an infection in her episiotomy
- **D.** hemorrhoids

_D_   **10.** The care Debbie receives in the recovery room should include
- **(1)** protection against infection
- **(2)** opportunity to rest
- **(3)** oral hygiene and perineal care
- **(4)** early detection of signs of complications
- **A.** (4) only
- **B.** (1) and (3)
- **C.** (2) and (4)
- **D.** All of these

_B_   **11.** Early ambulation is encouraged by some doctors following delivery. The advantages of early ambulation are that it helps
- **(1)** the mother regain her strength more rapidly
- **(2)** prevent circulatory problems
- **(3)** prevent bladder problems
- **(4)** the mother assume responsibility for her own care
- **A.** All of these
- **B.** All except (4)
- **C.** (1) only
- **D.** (2) and (3)

_A_   **12.** Before Debbie gets out of bed for the first time following delivery
- **(1)** there should be a doctor's order for it
- **(2)** her pads should be properly positioned to absorb the vaginal discharge
- **(3)** she should sit on the side of the bed for a few moments to regain her equilibrium
- **(4)** she should have a nurse with her
- **A.** All of these
- **B.** (1) and (4)
- **C.** (1), (2), and (3)
- **D.** (2), (3), and (4)

_C_   **13.** The important points in Debbie's bladder care would consist of
- **(1)** helping Debbie to the bathroom to urinate
- **(2)** catheterizing her every 8 to 12 hours
- **(3)** preventing overdistention of her bladder
- **(4)** making sure her bladder is emptied when she urinates
- **A.** (1) and (3)
- **B.** (2) and (4)
- **C.** (3) and (4)
- **D.** (2) and (3)

_B_   **14.** The daily measuring of the height of Debbie's fundus is done to find out
- **A.** if her bladder is distended
- **B.** the rate of involution
- **C.** if she has an infection
- **D.** if she is bleeding excessively

A   **15.** Which of the following findings would it be most important for you to report to the doctor if it were present on Debbie's third postpartum day?
  (1) cracked nipples
  (2) engorged breasts
  (3) fundus five fingerbreadths below the umbilicus
  (4) healing episiotomy
  A. (1) only
  B. (2) only
  C. (1) and (3)
  D. (2) and (4)

D   **16.** During the postpartum period, Debbie's diet should include additional
  (1) calories
  (2) proteins
  (3) minerals
  (4) vitamins
  A. None of these
  B. (2), (3), and (4)
  C. (1), (2), and (4)
  D. All of these

A   **17.** Debbie needs an abundant fluid intake during the postpartum period to
  (1) promote bladder function
  (2) promote bowel function
  (3) replace fluids lost during labor
  (4) replace fluid loss due to diuresis and diaphoresis
  A. All of these
  B. (1) and (3)
  C. (1) and (4)
  D. (2) and (4)

A   **18.** There are several advantages when the first bath Debbie receives following delivery is given by you. Some of these advantages are
  (1) she can express her feelings to you about her labor, the birth, and the baby
  (2) she can ask questions about the body changes and functions that are new to her
  (3) you can answer her questions and give her support and encouragement
  (4) you can instruct her in the proper care of her body at this time
  A. All of these
  B. (2) and (3)
  C. (1) and (2)
  D. (2) and (4)

C   **19.** When instructing Debbie concerning the care of her breasts, you would tell her that one of the best ways of preventing her nipples from becoming sore and cracked is to
  A. bathe her breasts with soap and water once a day
  B. apply ointment to her nipples following each feeding
  C. be sure that all of the nipple and as much as possible of the areola are in Jennifer's mouth when she nurses
  D. not permit Jennifer to nurse too long at each feeding until her milk comes in

B   **20.** Which of the following is *not* a hormone preparation used to suppress the action of prolactin in mothers who wish to formula-feed their infants?
  A. Deladumone
  B. Methergine
  C. Tace
  D. Stilbestrol

A   **21.** The measures that can be used to prevent infection in Debbie's episiotomy include
  (1) cleansing the area from front to back
  (2) attaching the pad in back first, then in front
  (3) thorough handwashing before touching the pad
  (4) avoid touching the side of the pad that is placed next to the stitches
  A. All except (2)
  B. All of these
  C. (1) and (3)
  D. (2) and (4)

_D_ 22. Debbie may experience several types of discomfort during the postpartum period. The doctor anticipates this and prescribes accordingly. If she complains of afterpains, which of the following that the doctor has prescribed for her comfort would be most appropriate to give her?
  A. heat lamp
  B. sitz bath
  C. sprays and ointments
  D. analgesics

_C_ 23. As far as exercises are concerned, the new mother
  (1) should not do any before the 6-week checkup
  (2) may do simple ones as soon as she feels like it
  (3) should start slowly and gradually increase to tolerance
  (4) should avoid fatigue
  (5) should not do strenuous ones until after the 6-week checkup
  A. (1) only
  B. all except (5)
  C. all except (1)
  D. (2), (3), and (4)

_B_ 24. An exercise Debbie could do to strengthen the perineal muscles is
  A. head raising
  B. Kegel
  C. stretching from head to toe
  D. lower back

_D_ 25. The exercise in question 24
  A. should not be done before the 6-week checkup
  B. should not be done after the 6-week checkup
  C. should be done in bed
  D. can be done anytime, anyplace

_A_ 26. It is recommended that a day or so after delivery, the labor and delivery nurse visit the new mother on the postpartum unit. The purpose of this visit is
  A. to help the mother assimilate her labor and delivery experience
  B. to renew the relationship between the nurse and mother
  C. so that the nurse can reassure the mother that she did well in labor and delivery
  D. so that the mother can thank the nurse for her help during labor and delivery

_D_ 27. The most important reason for the new mother to assimilate her labor and delivery experience is
  A. so that she can get on to the other postpartum tasks
  B. so that she can get her questions about the experience answered
  C. to clarify details of the experience
  D. to help prevent fear and anxiety in her next pregnancy

_B_ 28. The best way the postpartum nurse can help the new mother who is upset over her protruding abdomen is to
  A. tell her it is normal
  B. give her exercises and nutrition counseling
  C. tell her she will get her figure back if she breast-feeds her infant
  D. explain that it is due to the size of the baby she had

_A_ 29. Which of the following new mothers probably needs *most* help with mothering skills?
  A. a 35-year-old primipara who was an only child and who never babysat
  B. a 35-year-old multipara who was an only child and who never babysat
  C. an 18-year-old primipara who helped take care of four younger brothers and sisters
  D. an 18-year-old primipara who was an only child and who did a lot of babysitting of infants

_D_ 30. Probably the best way the nurse can help the new mother develop skill in caring for her new infant is to
  A. show the mother what to do for the baby
  B. tell the mother what to do for the baby
  C. praise the mother when she does well
  D. have the mother do the care after showing her how

_C_ **31.** The postpartum task that affects the woman's marital satisfaction has to do with
    A. her mothering skills
    B. relinquishing her fantasized infant and claiming the real infant
    C. redefining the relationship between herself and her husband
    D. her personal appearance

_A_ **32.** Which of the following are ways the postpartum nurse can help the new mother work through the postpartum tasks?
    (1) by stressing the importance of rest periods during the day
    (2) by being an interested listener
    (3) by helping both parents have realistic expectations of the mother when she goes home
    (4) by providing early and frequent contact with the infant
    (5) by giving her the phone number of the postpartum unit when she goes home
    A. All of these
    B. All except (1)
    C. (2), (3), and (4)
    D. All except (5)

_C_ **33.** If you discovered that Debbie had postpartum blues, you would
    (1) provide privacy
    (2) offer to stay with her a while if she desired
    (3) ignore it and leave her alone
    (4) assure her that this is a normal reaction
    A. All of these
    B. (1) and (2)
    C. (1), (2), and (4)
    D. (3) only

_C_ **34.** In teaching Debbie and Bob about sexual relations after childbirth you might tell them
    (1) to expect Debbie to have greater sexual desires for the first year
    (2) to use a water-soluble gel to decrease tightness and dryness of the vagina
    (3) to proceed cautiously at first because of tenderness and discomfort of the episiotomy
    (4) disruptions may occur
    (5) open communication is important
    A. (1) and (5)
    B. (2), (3), and (4)
    C. All except (1)
    D. All of these

_A_ **35.** Points to remember in order to make your teaching of patients effective include
    (1) first establishing a relationship of trust with the patient
    (2) finding out what the patient feels she needs to learn
    (3) speaking clearly and using terms the patient understands
    (4) having some means of testing the patient's understanding of what has been taught
    A. All of these
    B. (1), (2), and (3)
    C. (2) only
    D. (2) and (3)

II. Every morning during Debbie's postpartum hospital stay, you would examine her breasts, stitches and lochia to be sure physiological processes were occurring at a normal rate and that no pathologic processes were developing. Below is a list of things you would do in your exam. Number them (1, 2, 3 etc.) in the order that you should do them.

_8_ **A.** Inspect her lochia
_5_ **B.** Note the condition of her nipples
_3_ **C.** Wash your hands
_7_ **D.** Examine her episiotomy
_2_ **E.** Explain what you are going to do
_4_ **F.** Examine her breasts
_1_ **G.** Provide privacy
_6_ **H.** Measure the height of her fundus

III. In the space before the instruction you would give Debbie in Column I, place the letter of the reason why the instruction is given from Column II.

I INSTRUCTION	II REASON FOR THE INSTRUCTION
_E_ **1.** Drink plenty of water	**A.** Cleanliness
_D_ **2.** Increase intake of calories, proteins, minerals, and vitamins	**B.** Safety
_D_ **3.** Include at least a quart of milk in daily diet	**C.** Prevent infection
_B_ **4.** Have a nurse accompany her the first couple of times she gets out of bed and the first time she showers	**D.** Meet nutritional needs
_C_ **5.** Wash breasts first when taking a bath or shower	**E.** Promote body functions
_A_ **6.** Wear a clean bra each day	**F.** Derive greatest benefit
_F_ **7.** Apply nipple cream, sprays, and ointments as shown by nurse	
_C_ **8.** Wash hands thoroughly before and after changing perineal pad	
_C_ **9.** Do not touch the side of the pad that goes next to the episiotomy	
_B_ **10.** Resume ambulation and activities gradually	
_C_ **11.** Wash perineal area from front to back, never bring washcloth from anus back over stitches and vagina	

IV. In the space before the patient situation in Column I, place the letter of the step it describes in a nursing care plan, from Column II.

I PATIENT SITUATION	II STEPS IN A NURSING CARE PLAN
_A_ **1.** Observe patient's self-care. Ask her about her understanding of it.	**A.** Assessment
_D_ **2.** Demonstrates understanding of self-care	**B.** Potential Nursing Diagnosis
_B_ **3.** Knowledge deficit regarding self-care	**C.** Interventions
_C_ **4.** Teach patient self-care	**D.** Expected Outcome
_B_ **5.** Potential alteration in patterns of urinary elimination	
_C_ **6.** Encourage fluids	
_A_ **7.** Check rate of involution daily	
_D_ **8.** Involution occurs normally without complications	
_B_ **9.** Potential for injury or infection related to postpartum status	
_B_ **10.** Alterations in comfort: pain related to episiotomy or afterpains	
_A_ **11.** Observe parenting skills in interaction with infant	
_C_ **12.** Teach mother how to care for infant	
_D_ **13.** Discomfort is relieved	
_C_ **14.** Praise mother	
_B_ **15.** Potential alteration in parenting related to inexperience and feelings of inadequacy	

V. PROJECTS

1. Find out which medications to suppress lactation, with their dosage and frequency of administration, are prescribed most often by the doctors who practice obstetrics at your hospital.

    A. Medication   **B.** Dosage   **C.** Frequency of Administration

2. Find out what measures are taken by your hospital to provide family-centered maternity care.

    A. Rooming-in (What are the rules for it?)

    B. Sibling visitation

    C. Other measures

3. What are the visiting regulations for the maternity unit at your hospital? Are they for the patient's benefit or for the nurses' and doctors' convenience? Interview five postpartum patients and find out how they feel about them. Interview five nurses and/or doctors and find out how they feel about them. How do *you* feel about them? What changes would you make?

ANSWERS · CHAPTER 13

I.
  1. C
  2. A
  3. D
  4. B
  5. A
  6. A
  7. C
  8. D
  9. B

  10. D
  11. B
  12. A
  13. C
  14. B
  15. A
  16. D
  17. A
  18. A

  19. C
  20. B
  21. A
  22. D
  23. C
  24. B
  25. D
  26. A
  27. D

  28. B
  29. A
  30. D
  31. C
  32. A
  33. C
  34. C
  35. A

II.
  A. 8
  B. 5
  C. 3

  D. 7
  E. 2
  F. 4

  G. 1
  H. 6

III.
  1. E
  2. D
  3. D

  4. B
  5. C
  6. A

  7. F
  8. C
  9. C

  10. B
  11. C

IV.
  1. A
  2. D
  3. B
  4. C

  5. B
  6. C
  7. A
  8. D

  9. B
  10. B
  11. A
  12. C

  13. D
  14. C
  15. B

the normal newborn 14 at birth

I. SITUATION: One week past Debbie's estimated date of confinement, Debbie and Bob's first child, Jennifer, was born at 1:20 A.M. Jennifer cried spontaneously and lustily at birth and her color quickly changed to pink except for her hands and feet, which remained blue. She weighed 8 lb 1 oz (3,657 g) and her length was 21 inches. The circumference of her head was 14 inches while her chest was 13½ inches. She appeared to be healthy and normal.

Place the letter of the *best* answer in the space before the statement.

B   **1.** Compared to that of normal newborn infants, Jennifer's weight is
    A. below the normal range
    B. within the normal range
    C. a little above the normal range
    D. much above the normal range

D   **2.** If Bob had asked you about the white cheesy material in the creases of Jennifer's arms and legs, you could have explained that it protected her while she was in the "bag of waters" and that it is called
    A. molding
    B. lanugo
    C. caput succedaneum
    D. vernix caseosa

C   **3.** Debbie and Bob were both concerned about the elongated shape of Jennifer's head. You explain that this
    (1) is caused by overlapping of the skull bones during birth
    (2) is caused by hemorrhage into the space between the periosteum and the skull bone
    (3) is swelling caused by prolonged pressure on the head during labor
    (4) will disappear in a few hours without treatment
    A. All of these
    B. All except (3)
    C. All except (2)
    D. (4) only

B   **4.** Which of the following would you *not* expect Jennifer to have?
    A. flexed position
    B. coordinated movements
    C. fingernails
    D. eyebrows

A   **5.** When Debbie asked about the "soft spots" on Jennifer's head, you could explain that the anterior fontanel usually closes by the
    A. 18th month and the posterior by the 3rd month
    B. 3rd month and the posterior by the 18th month
    C. 12th month and the posterior by the 4th month
    D. 4th month and the posterior by the 12th month

C   **6.** Which of the following would *not* be true regarding Jennifer's eyes at birth?
     (1) they have their permanent color
     (2) tears are not produced when she cries
     (3) she can focus without difficulty
     (4) she can distinguish between light and dark and does not like bright lights
     A. (3) and (4)
     B. (2) and (3)
     C. (1) and (3)
     D. All of these

A   **7.** Debbie asks you when Jennifer's cord will come off. You can reply that usually the cord comes off in about
     A. 6 to 10 days
     B. 3 to 5 days
     C. 4 to 8 days
     D. 2 to 4 days

A   **8.** After the cord drops off, healing of the navel usually takes about
     A. a week
     B. a month
     C. 2 weeks
     D. 3 weeks

A   **9.** If Jennifer should become jaundiced on the second or third day after birth, you would suspect that it was due to
     A. destruction of excess red blood cells with the production of more bilirubin than her immature liver can handle
     B. her immature heat-regulating mechanism
     C. poor peripheral circulation
     D. deficient supply of the enzyme lipase

C   **10.** You would expect Jennifer to have her first stool within 8 to 10 hours after birth. This stool is
     A. yellow
     B. yellowish-green
     C. meconium
     D. transitional

B   **11.** You would prepare Debbie for Jennifer's physiologic weight loss by explaining that she will probably lose
     A. 2% to 3% of her birth weight
     B. 5% to 10% of her birth weight
     C. 10% to 15% of her birth weight
     D. 4% to 6% of her birth weight

D   **12.** Jennifer probably will regain her birth weight by the time she is
     A. 4 to 5 days old
     B. a week old
     C. a month old
     D. 10 to 14 days old

   13. Which of the following make it possible for Jennifer to obtain her food by sucking?
     (1) ridges in the roof of her mouth
     (2) fat pads inside her cheeks
     (3) strong sucking muscles
     (4) sucking reflex
     A. All of these
     B. (3) and (4)
     C. (1), (3), and (4)
     D. (2), (3), and (4)

D   **14.** While observing Jennifer sleeping, you noticed that her breathing was typical for a normal newborn. This means it was
     A. regular, quiet, and through her nose and chest
     B. irregular, noisy, and through her mouth and chest
     C. regular, noisy, and through her mouth and abdomen
     D. irregular, quiet, and through her nose and abdomen

B   **15.** You would expect Jennifer's respiratory rate to be about
- **A.** 10 to 15 per minute
- **B.** 35 to 50 per minute
- **C.** 15 to 20 per minute
- **D.** 25 to 30 per minute

C   **16.** You would expect Jennifer's pulse rate to be about
- **A.** 72 to 96 per minute
- **B.** 100 to 120 per minute
- **C.** 120 to 150 per minute
- **D.** 160 to 200 per minute

A   **17.** Factors which may have helped Jennifer to begin breathing at birth include
- **(1)** an increased amount of CO_2 for a brief time
- **(2)** an increased amount of CO_2 for a prolonged period
- **(3)** the change in temperature from the warm uterus to the cooler external environment
- **(4)** stimulation of her skin by the birth canal and the doctor's hands
- **A.** (1), (3) and (4)
- **B.** (2), (3), and (4)
- **C.** (1) and (4)
- **D.** (2) and (3)

C   **18.** When an object is placed in Jennifer's hand, she will take hold of it momentarily. This is a result of the
- **A.** Moro reflex
- **B.** cling reflex
- **C.** grasp reflex
- **D.** rooting reflex

D   **19.** The reflex that is employed in Jennifer's search for food is the
- **A.** Moro reflex
- **B.** sucking reflex
- **C.** swallowing reflex
- **D.** rooting reflex

A   **20.** The reflex that is employed when Jennifer responds to a loud noise or sudden movement of her crib by drawing up her legs and bringing her arms upward and forward is the
- **A.** Moro reflex
- **B.** Babinski reflex
- **C.** gag reflex
- **D.** cough reflex

B   **21.** Debbie can expect that, during the first weeks of life, Jennifer will sleep about
- **A.** 18 hours out of 24
- **B.** 20 hours out of 24
- **C.** 10 hours out of 24
- **D.** 12 hours out of 24

II. A. In the space before the term in Column I, place the letter of its definition from Column II.

I
TERM

II
DEFINITION

D 1. Caput succedaneum
G 2. Cephalhematoma
B 3. Circumcision
F 4. Erythematous blotches
H 5. Icterus neonatorum
A 6. Milia
C 7. Phimosis
I 8. Pseudomenstruation
E 9. "Stork bites"

A. Tiny white spots on the nose and forehead of some newborn infants

B. Surgical removal of the foreskin of the penis

C. Narrowness of opening of foreskin so that foreskin cannot be pulled back over glans

D. Swelling of the head of the newborn due to prolonged pressure by a partially dilated cervix

E. Small, deep pink areas of thin skin on eyelids, above nose, and on the nape of the neck of newborns

F. Large, red, hivelike areas on the skin of some newborns

G. Bleeding into the space between the skull bone and periosteum

H. Physiologic jaundice

I. Small bloody vaginal discharge 2 or 3 days after birth

B. In the space before the characteristic in Column I, place the letter or letters of the explanation for the characteristic from Column II.

I
CHARACTERISTICS OF
NORMAL NEWBORNS

II
EXPLANATION

D   1. Inability to focus eyes
M   2. Unstable temperature
K   3. Hands and feet cool to touch and bluish color first few hours
C   4. Large, flabby abdomen
N   5. Breast engorgement
F I P 6. Tendency to regurgitate feeding
L   7. Physiologic jaundice
A   8. Tearless crying
J Q   9. Ability to obtain food by sucking
E R   10. Initiation of respirations at birth
O   11. Inability to digest fat well
G   12. Physiologic weight loss
B   13. Reddish or rusty color on diaper following urination

A. Lacrimal glands do not function for several weeks after birth

B. Uric acid excreted in the urine

C. Size of abdominal organs and lack of tone of abdominal muscles

D. Lacks muscle coordination

E. Increase in CO_2 for brief period

F. Incompletely developed cardiac sphincter of stomach

G. Output exceeds intake

H. Hormone action on uterine lining before birth

I. Overfeeding and/or not burping adequately

J. Ridges in roof of mouth and sucking pads

K. Poor peripheral circulation

L. Destruction of excess red blood cells with production of more bilirubin than immature liver can manage

M. Immature heat-regulating mechanism

N. Effect of hormones produced by the placenta during pregnancy

O. Deficient supply of enzyme lipase

P. Result of swallowing discharges during birth

Q. Sucking reflex

R. Temperature change and skin stimulation

I. **1.** B   **7.** A   **12.** D   **17.** A
    2. D   **8.** A   **13.** A   **18.** C
    3. C   **9.** A   **14.** D   **19.** D
    4. B   **10.** C   **15.** B   **20.** A
    5. A   **11.** B   **16.** C   **21.** B
    6. C

II. **A.** **1.** D   **4.** F   **7.** C
       2. G   **5.** H   **8.** I
       3. B   **6.** A   **9.** E

    B. **1.** D   **5.** N   **8.** A   **11.** O
       2. M   **6.** F, I, P   **9.** J, Q   **12.** G
       3. K   **7.** L   **10.** E, R   **13.** B
       4. C

nursing care of the 15 newborn

I. SITUATION: As soon as Jennifer's head was born the doctor suctioned her nose and mouth. As the rest of her body was born, Jennifer began to cry lustily. The doctor spoke softly and held her securely as he again suctioned her mouth and nose while keeping her head lower than her body. Jennifer showed her displeasure at being suctioned by crying and moving her arms and legs. As soon as he was sure he had cleared her airway, the doctor stopped suctioning her and held her upright for her parents to see. Jennifer stopped crying and began looking around. Within 1 minute after birth she was pink, except for her hands and feet, which were blue. After her cord stopped pulsating, the doctor clamped and cut it. Then he placed Jennifer on the warm, sterile receiving blanket in the heated crib. The nurse quickly and thoroughly wiped Jennifer dry, including her head. She then weighed her and placed her in the heated crib and wrapped her snugly in a warm, dry blanket. After wrapping her in a second blanket, the nurse offered her to her daddy, Bob, to hold. The nurse proceeded to make the identification bracelets for Jennifer and her mother, Debbie, and to complete the charting. As soon as the doctor finished repairing the episiotomy and Debbie was positioned comfortably, she held Jennifer and both parents inspected this first new member of the family. Debbie decided she would like to nurse Jennifer before she was taken to the nursery, so the nurse and Bob helped her do so. Jennifer wasn't too cooperative at first but after a few tries she took hold of the nipple and began to nurse, much to everyone's delight. When Debbie and Bob were ready, the nurse took Jennifer and applied identification bracelets and the prophylactic eye medication. Then she obtained Jennifer's footprints and Debbie's thumbprints. Finally, Jennifer was taken to the nursery.

Place the letter of the *best* answer in the space before the statement.

_B_   **1.** The doctor suctioned Jennifer's nose and mouth as soon as her head was born to
     (1) prevent hemorrhage
     (2) clear her airway
     (3) prevent aspiration of fluid and mucus
     (4) prevent cold stress
     A. (1) and (2)
     B. (2) and (3)
     C. (3) and (4)
     D. (4) only

_A_   **2.** The doctor clamped Jennifer's umbilical cord to
     (1) prevent hemorrhage
     (2) promote healing
     (3) prevent infection
     (4) help it dry so it will drop off sooner
     A. (1) only
     B. (2) and (3)
     C. (1) and (4)
     D. All of these

_D_   **3.** The doctor waited until Jennifer's cord stopped pulsating before he clamped it to
     A. prevent hemorrhage
     B. decrease her blood volume by 50 to 100 ml
     C. drain it so it will dry and drop off more quickly
     D. increase her blood volume by 50 to 100 ml

_C_ **4.** The nurse wiped Jennifer dry to
   A. stimulate her to cry
   B. stimulate her circulation
   C. prevent cold stress
   D. make her feel more comfortable

_A_ **5.** The Apgar score Jennifer should receive 1 minute after birth is
   A. 9
   B. 10
   C. 8
   D. 7

_D_ **6.** You would give Jennifer the lowest score for
   A. heart rate
   B. respiratory effort
   C. reflex irritability
   D. color

_C_ **7.** Problems Jennifer could have as a result of cold stress include
   (1) apnea
   (2) hypoglycemia
   (3) acidosis
   (4) respiratory distress syndrome
   A. (1) and (3)
   B. (2) and (4)
   C. All of these
   D. None of these

_B_ **8.** Jennifer was placed in a heated crib to prevent heat loss by
   A. evaporation
   B. conduction
   C. convection
   D. radiation

_A_ **9.** In order to prevent Jennifer from getting cold while her parents get acquainted with her, you should
   A. first wrap her snugly in a warm blanket, except for her face, before letting them hold her
   B. keep her in the heated crib but uncover her so that they can inspect her
   C. take her directly to the nursery and let her parents see her through the nursery window
   D. take her directly to the nursery and wait until her temperature is stabilized before taking her to her parents

In the nursery, Jennifer was placed in an incubator and her temperature was taken. After about 3 hours she was given a bath and dressed and placed in a crib in the nursery.

_C_ **10.** While Jennifer was in the incubator, you would check her temperature and the temperature of the incubator every hour to
   (1) see if her temperature is stable
   (2) see if her temperature is within the desired range
   (3) avoid overheating her
   (4) see if the incubator is working properly
   A. (1) only
   B. (2) and (4)
   C. (2) and (3)
   D. (4) only

_D_ **11.** Safety measures that you would employ when weighing Jennifer include
   (1) locating the scale in a warm part of the room, away from drafts and outside windows
   (2) covering the scale with a warm paper or towel
   (3) keeping your hand above Jennifer while she is on the scale
   (4) completing the procedure as quickly as possible
   A. (1) only
   B. (2) and (3)
   C. All except (4)
   D. All of these

_C_ **12.** Measures that can be taken to minimize heat loss during Jennifer's bath include
- **(1)** keeping her wrapped except for the part that is being bathed
- **(2)** drying each part thoroughly and covering it as soon as it is bathed
- **(3)** using cotton balls and a mild soap
- **(4)** using a radiant heat warmer during the bath
- **A.** (1) only
- **B.** (2) and (4)
- **C.** All except (3)
- **D.** All of these

_B_ **13.** Which of the following observations should be made of Jennifer during the first hours after birth?
- **(1)** inspecting her cord for bleeding
- **(2)** observing for mucus
- **(3)** noting her color and respirations
- **(4)** noting and recording her first voiding and first stool
- **A.** (1) and (2)
- **B.** All of these
- **C.** All except (4)
- **D.** (2) and (3)

_B_ **14.** If Jennifer had a lot of mucus, the best way to promote drainage of it would be to position her on her
- **A.** back with the crib flat
- **B.** side with the head of the crib lowered
- **C.** side with the head of the crib elevated
- **D.** back with the head of the crib elevated

_A_ **15.** Measures you could take while caring for Jennifer to protect her against infection include
- **(1)** thorough handwashing before and after caring for her
- **(2)** keeping your fingernails short and free of polish
- **(3)** not caring for her if you have an infection
- **(4)** providing her with her own supplies and equipment in the drawer of her crib
- **A.** All of these
- **B.** All except (2)
- **C.** (1) and (3)
- **D.** (3) and (4)

Debbie has rooming-in after Jennifer is 24 hours old. You are assigned to care for mother and baby and, as part of your responsibility, you wish to assist Debbie in developing her mothering skills. This includes teaching her how to bathe Jennifer.

_C_ **16.** You could tell Debbie that the *least* desirable time for Jennifer's bath is
- **A.** at bedtime
- **B.** early in the morning
- **C.** right after a feeding
- **D.** just before a feeding

_B_ **17.** The most important safety precaution Debbie should take while giving Jennifer her bath is to
- **A.** remove her jewelry, which might scratch Jennifer
- **B.** never leave Jennifer alone on the table or in the tub
- **C.** place a washcloth or diaper on the bottom of the tub
- **D.** avoid extremes in temperature of the bath water

_D_ **18.** Special instructions you could give Debbie concerning Jennifer's bath could include
- **(1)** how to get into Jennifer's neck crease
- **(2)** the importance of bathing, rinsing well, and thoroughly drying all creases
- **(3)** how to bathe her genitalia
- **(4)** how to apply powder and oil
- **A.** (3) only
- **B.** (1) and (2)
- **C.** All except (4)
- **D.** All of these

_A_ **19.** Jennifer should not be given a tub bath until
- **A.** her cord is off and her navel is healed
- **B.** she can sit alone
- **C.** she is used to being bathed and enjoys it
- **D.** her temperature is stable

_C_ **20.** The care of Jennifer's cord includes
   (1) prevention of infection
   (2) prevention of irritation
   (3) keeping it dry
   (4) keeping it covered with a moist dressing
   A. (4) only
   B. (1), (2), and (4)
   C. (1), (2), and (3)
   D. (1) and (3)

_B_ **21.** The clothing Jennifer will wear while she is in the hospital probably will consist of a
   (1) shirt
   (2) diaper
   (3) gown
   (4) dress
   A. (1), (2), and (3)
   B. (1) and (2)
   C. (2) and (3)
   D. (1), (2), and (4)

_D_ **22.** The care of an infant during the first few hours following a circumcision includes
   (1) administering medication for pain
   (2) observing for hemorrhage
   (3) observing to see if he can urinate
   (4) applying petrolatum jelly on a square of gauze to the penis
   A. All of these
   B. (1) and (2)
   C. (2) and (3)
   D. (2) and (4)

_B_ **23.** The decision to have, or not to have, an infant circumcised is the responsibility of the
   A. obstetrician
   B. parents
   C. nurse
   D. pediatrician

_C_ **24.** Suggestions you can make to help Debbie avoid sore nipples include
   (1) nursing Jennifer as soon as possible after she is born
   (2) nursing Jennifer on a "demand" schedule
   (3) nursing Jennifer 5 to 7 minutes on each breast at each feeding until her milk comes in
   (4) putting all of her nipple and as much as possible of the areola into Jennifer's mouth when she nurses
   A. All of these
   B. (1) and (2)
   C. (3) and (4)
   D. (2) and (3)

Although Debbie is breast-feeding Jennifer, she wishes to learn how to prepare formula because she plans to return to work in a few weeks. You teach her:

_A_ **25.** Commonly used ingredients of formula are
   (1) water
   (2) carbohydrate
   (3) evaporated milk
   (4) whole milk
   A. (1), (2), and (3)
   B. (1) and (4)
   C. (2) and (4)
   D. (1) and (3)

_C_ **26.** Which of the following recipes for formula would contain the *least* amount of water?
   A. 1:2 E.M., 1 T dark Karo
   B. 1:3 E.M., 1 T dark Karo
   C. 1:1 E.M., 1 T dark Karo
   D. all of them contain the same amount of water

_B_ 27. Which of the following statements apply to the aseptic method of formula preparation?
    (1) all the supplies are washed and sterilized first
    (2) sterilization is accomplished by boiling for 5 minutes
    (3) sterilization is accomplished by boiling for 25 minutes
    (4) this method is convenient when only one or two bottles of formula are needed
    A. (1), (3), and (4)
    B. (1), (2), and (4)
    C. (2) and (4)
    D. (1) and (4)

_A_ 28. Suggestions you could give Debbie to avoid breakage of bottles when she uses the terminal method of formula preparation include
    (1) tightening the nipple caps before the bottles are put into the sterilizer
    (2) placing a cloth on the bottom of the sterilizer if no rack is available
    (3) adding another 2 inches of water to the sterilizer after water has boiled for 25 minutes
    (4) loosening the nipple caps before the bottles are put into the sterilizer
    A. (2) and (4)
    B. (3) and (4)
    C. (1) and (3)
    D. (1) and (2)

_D_ 29. Debbie can prevent scum formation, which could clog the nipples, by
    A. removing bottles from sterilizer as soon as the sterilization is done
    B. removing the lid from the sterilizer after the water begins to boil
    C. removing the nipples from the bottles as soon as the sterilization is done
    D. waiting until the sides of the sterilizer are cool enough to be handled before lifting the lid

_B_ 30. Measures that Debbie can take to lessen the chance of Jennifer's becoming ill as a result of bacterial growth in the formula include
    (1) refrigerating the formula following sterilization
    (2) discarding unused portions after each feeding
    (3) rinsing bottles and nipples with cold water immediately after each feeding
    (4) keeping the nipple on the formula bottle covered until ready for use
    A. All of these
    B. (1), (2), and (4)
    C. (1) and (2)
    D. (2), (3), and (4)

_C_ 31. Which of the following would be an effective way to meet the emotional needs of a formula-fed infant?
    A. diaper the infant before the feeding
    B. tilt the bottle so that milk fills the nipple during the feeding
    C. hold the infant while feeding
    D. burp the infant before, during, and after the feeding

II. Complete the following nursing care plan for a newborn infant by selecting from the list below the potential nursing diagnoses, nursing interventions, and expected outcomes for the assessments that are given and writing them under the correct heading.

ASSESSMENTS	POTENTIAL NURSING DIAGNOSES	INTERVENTIONS	EXPECTED OUTCOME
Observe breathing			
Take temperature; observe color			
Note physical appearance			
Take vital signs; determine gestational age; note neurological development; weigh; measure length and head circumference			
Observe behavioral pattern: sleep and activity, responsiveness			
Inspect cord and circumcision (male infants)			
Determine well-being of infant			
Observe for first and subsequent stools and urination			
Observe parent-infant interaction			

Provide opportunity for parents to hold and get acquainted with infant

Potential for infection related to newborn status and lack of normal skin flora

Record color, consistency, and amount of all stools

Parents are comfortable with infant and confident in caring for him

Position on side

Impaired gas exchange related to cold stress

Change position frequently

Ineffective breathing patterns related to obstructed airway

Report bleeding from cord or circumcision

Avoid drafts when bathing

Report if no urination occurs in first 24 hours

Record number of wet diapers

Positive interaction

Potential for injury, infection, or bleeding related to cord or circumcision

Infant is comfortable

Record temperature of warmer frequently

Suction as necessary

Potential impairment of skin integrity related to lack of normal flora* and peeling and cracking of skin

Wash hands before and after caring for each infant

Apply vaseline to circumcision to keep diaper from sticking to it

Urinates within first 24 hours and about 6 to 10 times every 24 hours

Infant is warm and temperature becomes stable

Intact skin

Cleanse cord with anti-infective agent according to hospital policy

Use individual technique†

Wrap warmly after bath

Minimum loss of birth weight, gains weight steadily

Neurological development consistent with gestational age

Stimulate infant through touch, sound, eye contact

Altered growth and development related to preterm or post-term status, SGA, or LGA

Alteration in patterns of urinary elimination related to insufficient fluid intake

Cold stress is avoided, color is normal

Report if no stool occurs in first 24 hours

No bleeding or infection

Breathes normally

Place in warmer

Change diaper as necessary

Alterations in comfort: pain related to wet diaper, position, hunger, circumcision

Reclamp cord if bleeding occurs

Bathe when temperature is stable

Assist parents as necessary, stay in background when not needed

Report if number of wet diapers decreases

Alterations in bowel elimination related to imperforate anus

Infant responds to stimulation, alternates sleep and activity

Tilt head of crib as necessary to promote drainage

Has meconium within first 24 hours

Infant adjusts to extrauterine life without problems

Feed when hungry

Potential alterations in parenting related to inexperience and feelings of inadequacy

Potential alteration in body temperature related to birth and newborn status

No infection

Keep bulb syringe in crib

Hold infant, encourage parents to hold and cuddle infant

Report bleeding from cord or circumcision

Record temperature on appropriate forms

Record assessments, report abnormals, graph weight daily, adjust feedings to promote appropriate growth

Impaired adjustment to extrauterine life related to preterm or post-term status or to other conditions such as malformations

Allow quiet time for sleep

Prevent skin breakdown by gentle handling, and changing diapers when wet or soiled

---

*Microorganisms that normally live in different parts of the body (skin, mouth, gastrointestinal tract, respiratory tract) and are usually harmless to the part of the body where they reside, are referred to as "normal flora." These organisms are helpful in preventing infection by pathogenic microorganisms.

†Individual technique involves perceiving each infant as an individual with needs specific to him and then tailoring the nursing interventions to meet these needs. It includes providing him with his own supplies and equipment, keeping his crib the recommended distance from cribs of other infants, and using aseptic technique to prevent infections.

I.

1. B	**9.** A	**17.** B	**25.** A
2. A	**10.** C	**18.** D	**26.** C
3. D	**11.** D	**19.** A	**27.** B
4. C	**12.** C	**20.** C	**28.** A
5. A	**13.** B	**21.** B	**29.** D
6. D	**14.** B	**22.** D	**30.** B
7. C	**15.** A	**23.** B	**31.** C
8. B	**16.** C	**24.** C	

II.

ASSESSMENTS	POTENTIAL NURSING DIAGNOSES	INTERVENTIONS	EXPECTED OUTCOME
Observe breathing	Ineffective breathing patterns related to obstructed airway	Position on one side; suction as necessary; tilt head of crib as necessary to promote drainage; keep bulb syringe in crib	Breathes normally
Take temperature; observe color	Potential alteration in body temperature related to birth and newborn status	Place in warmer; record temperature on appropriate forms; record temperature of warmer frequently	Infant is warm and temperature becomes stable
	Impaired gas exchange related to cold stress	Bathe when temperature is stable; avoid drafts when bathing; wrap warmly after bath	Cold stress is avoided; color is normal
Note physical appearance	Potential for infection related to newborn status and lack of normal skin flora	Wash hands before and after caring for each infant; use individual technique	No infection
	Potential impairment of skin integrity related to lack of normal flora and peeling and cracking of skin	Prevent skin breakdown by gentle handling and changing diapers when wet or soiled	Intact skin
Take vital signs; determine gestational age; note neurological development; weigh; measure length and head circumference	Altered growth and development related to preterm or post-term status, SGA, or LGA	Record assessments, report abnormals, graph weight daily, adjust feedings to promote appropriate growth	Minimum loss of birth weight, gains weight steadily, neurolgical development consistent with gestational age
Observe behavioral pattern: sleep and activity, responsiveness	Impaired adjustment to extrauterine life related to preterm or post-term status or to other conditions such as malformations	Stimulate infant through touch, sound, eye contact; allow quiet time for sleep	Infant adjusts to extrauterine life without problems; infant responds to stimulation; alternates sleep and activity
Inspect cord and circumcision (male infants)	Potential for injury, infection, or bleeding related to cord or circumcision	Cleanse cord with anti-infective agent according to hospital policy; reclamp cord if bleeding occurs; report bleeding from cord or circumcision	No bleeding or infection

ASSESSMENTS	POTENTIAL NURSING DIAGNOSES	INTERVENTIONS	EXPECTED OUTCOME
Determine well-being of infant	Alterations in comfort: pain related to wet diaper, position, hunger, circumcision	Change diaper as necessary; change position frequently; feed when hungry; hold infant, encourage parents to hold and cuddle infant; apply vaseline to circumcision to keep diaper from sticking to it	Infant is comfortable
Observe for first and subsequent stools and urination	Alterations in bowel elimination related to imperforate anus	Record color, consistency, and amount of all stools; report if no stool occurs in first 24 hours	Has meconium within first 24 hours
	Alteration in patterns of urinary elimination related to insufficient fluid intake	Record number of wet diapers; report if no urination occurs in first 24 hours; report if number of wet diapers decreases	Urinates within first 24 hours and about 6 to 10 times every 24 hours
Observe parent-infant interaction	Potential alterations in parenting related to inexperience and feelings of inadequacy	Provide opportunity for parents to hold and get acquainted with infant; assist parents as necessary, stay in background when not needed	Parents are comfortable with infant and confident in caring for him; positive interaction

health problems during 16 pregnancy

I. Place the letter of the *best* answer in the space before the statement.

_____ C **1.** When a woman dies as a result of a complication of childbirth, her death is classified as a
    A. neonatal mortality
    B. fetal mortality
    C. maternal mortality
    D. infant mortality

_____ B **2.** The most frequent causes of hemorrhage during the first half of pregnancy are
    A. placenta previa and abruptio placentae
    B. abortions and ectopic pregnancies
    C. abortions and placenta previa
    D. ectopic pregnancies and abruptio placentae

_____ D **3.** The most frequent causes of hemorrhage during the last half of pregnancy are
    A. ectopic pregnancies and abruptio placentae
    B. abortions and ectopic pregnancies
    C. abortions and placenta previa
    D. placenta previa and abruptio placentae

_____ A **4.** Termination of pregnancy before the age of viability without mechanical or medical interference is called
    A. spontaneous abortion
    B. criminal abortion
    C. induced abortion
    D. therapeutic abortion

_____ C **5.** Deliberate, intentional termination of pregnancy, without medical indications, before the age of viability is called
    A. spontaneous abortion
    B. criminal abortion
    C. induced abortion
    D. therapeutic abortion

_____ D **6.** Termination of pregnancy before the age of viability using medical means in an accredited medical facility is called
    A. spontaneous abortion
    B. criminal abortion
    C. induced abortion
    D. legal abortion

_____ B **7.** When a patient early in pregnancy experiences bleeding, with or without cramps or backache, the condition is called
    A. an inevitable abortion
    B. a threatened abortion
    C. a complete abortion
    D. an incomplete abortion

_A_ 8. When the bleeding and cramps are accompanied by rupture of the membranes and dilatation of the cervix, the condition is called
   A. an inevitable abortion
   B. a threatened abortion
   C. a complete abortion
   D. an incomplete abortion

_D_ 9. When parts of the products of conception are expelled and parts are retained, the type of abortion is
   A. an inevitable abortion
   B. a threatened abortion
   C. a complete abortion
   D. an incomplete abortion

_C_ 10. When all the products of conception are expelled, the type of abortion is
   A. an inevitable abortion
   B. a threatened abortion
   C. a complete abortion
   D. an incomplete abortion

_A_ 11. When a woman has three or more consecutive, spontaneous abortions, the condition is known as
   A. habitual abortion
   B. incompetent cervix
   C. missed abortion
   D. hydatidiform mole

_C_ 12. When the fetus dies but is retained for 2 months or longer before being expelled, the condition is known as
   A. habitual abortion
   B. incompetent cervix
   C. missed abortion
   D. hydatidiform mole

_B_ 13. When dilatation occurs as a result of the weight of the fetus, usually between the fourth and sixth month of pregnancy, the condition is known as
   A. habitual abortion
   B. incompetent cervix
   C. missed abortion
   D. hydatidiform mole

_D_ 14. A benign neoplasm of the chorion, in which the chorionic villi become filled with a clear, viscid fluid and resemble a cluster of grapes, is known as
   A. incompetent cervix
   B. ectopic pregnancy
   C. choriocarcinoma
   D. hydatidiform mole

_D_ 15. Follow-up care of hydatidiform mole consists of
   (1) tests to detect choriocarcinoma
   (2) chest x-rays
   (3) determining the amount of chorionic gonadotropin in the serum
   (4) advising the woman against becoming pregnant for a while
   A. (1), (2), and (3)
   B. (2), (3), and (4)
   C. (1), (3), and (4)
   D. All of these

_C_ 16. Most ectopic pregnancies occur in the
   A. abdominal cavity
   B. cervix
   C. fallopian tubes
   D. ovaries

_B_ 17. Which of the following may be used to diagnose ectopic pregnancy?
   (1) beta HCG
   (2) ultrasound
   (3) culdocentesis
   (4) laparoscopy
   (5) linear salpingostomy
   A. (1), (4), and (5)
   B. All except (5)
   C. All of these
   D. (2), (3), and (5)

A **18.** The treatment for ectopic pregnancy may include
- **(1)** linear salpingostomy
- **(2)** chest x-ray
- **(3)** antibiotics
- **(4)** blood transfusions
- **A.** (1) and (4)
- **B.** (2) and (3)
- **C.** All of these
- **D.** All except (3)

C **19.** Potential nursing diagnoses for a patient with an ectopic pregnancy may include
- **(1)** knowledge deficit related to her condition
- **(2)** potential for injury, weakness, shock related to blood loss
- **(3)** grief related to loss of pregnancy
- **(4)** anxiety related to future fertility
- **A.** (1) and (4)
- **B.** (2) and (3)
- **C.** All of these
- **D.** All except (2)

A **20.** A condition in which the placenta is located near the internal os of the cervix is known as
- **A.** placenta previa
- **B.** abruptio placentae
- **C.** pregnancy-induced hypertension (PIH)
- **D.** hyperemesis gravidarum

C **21.** The characteristic symptom of placenta previa is
- **A.** sudden, sharp, stabbing abdominal pain
- **B.** concealed bleeding
- **C.** painless bleeding
- **D.** rigid uterus; tender, painful abdomen

A **22.** Probably the safest and most accurate method of locating the placenta during pregnancy is by
- **A.** ultrasound
- **B.** arteriogram
- **C.** vaginal exam
- **D.** abdominal palpation

B **23.** Premature separation of a normally implanted placenta is known as
- **A.** placenta previa
- **B.** abruptio placentae
- **C.** PIH
- **D.** hyperemesis gravidarum

B **24.** Symptoms of abruptio placentae might include
- **(1)** sudden, sharp, stabbing abdominal pain
- **(2)** concealed bleeding
- **(3)** painless bleeding
- **(4)** rigid uterus; tender, painful abdomen
- **A.** (1) and (2)
- **B.** (2) and (4)
- **C.** (1) and (3)
- **D.** (1) only

A **25.** Which of the following is *not* included in the nursing care of an expectant mother who is admitted to the hospital because of bleeding?
- **A.** examine to find out the dilatation of the cervix
- **B.** observe for bleeding
- **C.** listen to fetal heart tones and take mother's blood pressure
- **D.** be sensitive to the mother's feelings

D **26.** Disseminated intravascular coagulation (DIC) is a life-threatening condition in which
- **A.** there is a problem with the location of the placenta
- **B.** there is a problem with the attachment of the placenta
- **C.** the blood clots too rapidly
- **D.** the blood does not clot

_B_ **27.** DIC is most often associated with
   A. placenta previa
   B. premature separation of the placenta
   C. septic abortion
   D. missed abortion when the fetus is retained for 5 weeks or longer

_D_ **28.** The leading cause of death among newborn infants during the first 4 weeks of life is
   A. congenital abnormalities
   B. pregnancy-induced hypertension
   C. hemorrhage during pregnancy
   D. premature birth

_B_ **29.** Another term for hyperemesis gravidarum is
   A. PIH
   B. pernicious vomiting
   C. preeclampsia
   D. eclampsia

_D_ **30.** In caring for the patient with hyperemesis gravidarum, the nurse should
   (1) be cheerful and optimistic
   (2) make sure the food served is neither hot nor cold
   (3) discuss the foods with the patient before serving them
   (4) place the emesis basin on the tray with the food when it is served
   A. All of these
   B. (1) and (3)
   C. (2) and (4)
   D. (1) only

_B_ **31.** PIH (toxemia) occurs most often in
   A. older multigravidae
   B. young primigravidae
   C. young multigravidae
   D. older primigravidae

_C_ **32.** PIH (toxemia) usually occurs after the
   A. 16th week of pregnancy
   B. 20th week of pregnancy
   C. 24th week of pregnancy
   D. 34th week of pregnancy

_D_ **33.** Which of the following changes in blood pressures during pregnancy would be considered a symptom of PIH?
   (1) a drop of 30 mm or more in the systolic or of 15 mm or more in the diastolic below the normal levels for the individual mother
   (2) a rise of 30 mm or more in the systolic or of 15 mm or more in the diastolic above the normal levels for the individual mother
   (3) a blood pressure of 130/90 or higher in any pregnant woman
   (4) a blood pressure of 140/90 in a pregnant woman whose blood pressure is usually 120/70
   A. (1) and (4)
   B. (2) only
   C. (3) only
   D. (2) and (4)

_B_ **34.** A sudden, excessive weight gain usually means
   A. the mother is overeating
   B. the mother is retaining fluid in her tissues
   C. the mother is not getting sufficient exercise
   D. the fetus is putting on fat

_A_ **35.** Often the first indication of swelling the expectant mother notices is when her
   A. rings become too tight
   B. shoes become too tight
   C. eyelids become puffy
   D. ankle bones are no longer distinguishable

_D_ **36.** Which of the following is *not* a symptom of preeclampsia?
   A. hypertension
   B. edema
   C. albuminuria
   D. convulsions and coma

_C_ **37.** Which of the following are symptoms of eclampsia?
  (1) hypertension
  (2) edema
  (3) albuminuria
  (4) convulsions and coma
  A. (1), (2), and (3)
  B. (2), (3), and (4)
  C. All of these
  D. (4) only

_D_ **38.** Signs that might indicate that the preeclamptic patient is about to have a convulsion include
  (1) epigastric pain
  (2) hypotension
  (3) visual disturbances
  (4) headache
  A. All of these
  B. (1), (2), and (3)
  C. (2), (3), and (4)
  D. (1), (3), and (4)

_A_ **39.** Nursing care of a mother with preeclampsia includes
  (1) carrying out the doctor's orders carefully
  (2) providing an environment favorable for rest and sleep
  (3) observing the mother closely for signs of impending convulsions
  (4) listening to the fetal heart tones and observing the mother for labor
  A. All of these
  B. (1) only
  C. (2), (3), and (4)
  D. All except (4)

_B_ **40.** Following delivery, the symptoms of PIH
  A. continue as before
  B. gradually disappear
  C. immediately disappear
  D. become more severe

_D_ **41.** The expectant mother who is Rh-negative is classified as
  A. heterozygous recessive
  B. heterozygous dominant
  C. homozygous dominant
  D. homozygous recessive

_B_ **42.** When an Rh-negative woman is married to an Rh-negative man, it would be expected that
  A. their children would be Rh-positive
  B. their children would be Rh-negative
  C. half of their children would be Rh-negative and half Rh-positive
  D. some of their children would develop Rh incompatibility

_C_ **43.** The only time there is a possibility of a problem due to Rh incompatibility is when
  A. an Rh-positive woman married to an Rh-negative man gives birth to an Rh-negative child
  B. an Rh-positive woman married to an Rh-negative man gives birth to an Rh-positive child
  C. an Rh-negative woman married to an Rh-positive man gives birth to an Rh-positive child
  D. an Rh-negative woman married to an Rh-positive man gives birth to an Rh-negative child

_A_ **44.** An antibody titer test is done on the Rh-negative mother during pregnancy to find out if
  A. the mother is producing antibodies against Rh-positive blood cells at a rapid rate
  B. the mother is producing antibodies against Rh-negative blood cells at a rapid rate
  C. the fetus is producing antibodies against Rh-positive blood cells at a rapid rate
  D. the fetus is producing antibodies against Rh-negative blood cells at a rapid rate

_D_ **45.** Rh incompatibility may result in
   (1) destruction of fetal red blood cells
   (2) anemia of the fetus
   (3) erythroblastosis fetalis
   A. None of these
   B. All except (1)
   C. (2) and (3)
   D. All of these

_B_ **46.** When amniocentesis reveals that the fetus is being severely affected by Rh incompatibility but is too immature to survive outside the uterus, it might be possible to treat the fetus by giving
   A. Rho (D) immune globulin to the mother
   B. a transfusion to the fetus
   C. Rho (D) immune globulin to the fetus
   D. a transfusion to the mother

_C_ **47.** Rho (D) immune globulin is an immune globulin which acts by combining with, and thus neutralizing, any Rh-positive red blood cells which have crossed from the fetal circulation to the maternal circulation. To be effective, it must be given
   (1) to sensitized Rh-negative women
   (2) within 72 hours after delivery
   (3) after each pregnancy in which an Rh-positive infant is born to an unsensitized Rh-negative mother
   (4) to unsensitized Rh-negative women following abortions, ectopic pregnancies, and stillbirths
   A. All of these
   B. All except (4)
   C. All except (1)
   D. All except (3)

_A_ **48.** The usual dosage of Rho (D) immune globulin is
   A. 1 ml intramuscularly
   B. 2 ml intramuscularly
   C. 1 ml orally
   D. 2 ml orally

_B_ **49.** Patients whose diabetes is first discovered during pregnancy are known as
   A. pregestational diabetics
   B. gestational diabetics
   C. juvenile diabetics
   D. adult diabetics

_B_ **50.** After the first 2 or 3 months of pregnancy, the diabetic's insulin requirements usually
   A. decrease slightly
   B. increase
   C. remain the same
   D. decrease greatly

_D_ **51.** Factors which must be considered when planning the diet of the pregnant diabetic include the
   (1) nutritional needs of mother and fetus
   (2) importance of keeping the diabetes under control
   (3) mother's weight
   (4) mother's activities
   A. (1) and (2)
   B. (1) and (4)
   C. (2) and (3)
   D. All of these

_B_ **52.** The most important factors in determining the effect diabetes has on pregnancy seem to be
   (1) the age and health of the mother
   (2) how well controlled the diabetes is
   (3) the number of past pregnancies the mother has had
   (4) the length of time the mother has had diabetes
   A. (1) and (3)
   B. (2) and (4)
   C. All except (3)
   D. All of these

_C_ **53.** Uncontrolled diabetes may affect pregnancy by causing
    (1) fetal death due to placental insufficiency
    (2) fetal death due to fetal acidosis resulting from maternal ketosis
    (3) an increase in such complications as PIH and hydramnios
    (4) an increase in the number of infants born with congenital anomalies
    A. (1) and (2)
    B. (3) and (4)
    C. All of these
    D. None of these

_B_ **54.** Tests which may be done to determine the well-being of the fetus of a diabetic mother include
    (1) L/S ratio determination
    (2) oxytocin challenge test
    (3) determination of maternal estriol levels
    (4) roll-over tests
    A. (1) and (4)
    B. (1), (2) and (3)
    C. (1) and (2)
    D. (2) and (4)

_C_ **55.** Which of the following accounts for approximately 15% of all perinatal deaths?
    A. placenta previa
    B. myomas
    C. premature separation of the placenta
    D. ectopic pregnancy

_A_ **56.** The most prevalent type of heart disease among pregnant women is
    A. congenital heart disease
    B. mitral valve insufficiency
    C. aortic stenosis
    D. pericarditis

_C_ **57.** A viral disease which causes only mild symptoms in the mother but may result in congenital malformations in the fetus if the mother gets it during the first 12 weeks of pregnancy is
    A. syphilis
    B. gonorrhea
    C. rubella
    D. rubeola

_B_ **58.** The newborn infant may become blind, unless preventive treatment is given, if the mother has
    A. syphilis
    B. gonorrhea
    C. rubella
    D. rubeola

_B_ **59.** Mechanical blockage of the fallopian tubes resulting in sterility may be caused by
    A. syphilis
    B. gonorrhea
    C. rubella
    D. rubeola

_C_ **60.** One of the newer sexually transmitted diseases is
    A. syphilis
    B. gonorrhea
    C. AIDS
    D. PIH

_B_ **61.** The most devastating effect of the disease in question 60 is that it
    A. causes mechanical blockage of the fallopian tubes
    B. destroys the body's immune system
    C. causes blindness in the newborns of untreated mothers
    D. results in congenital malformations in newborns of untreated mothers

_D_ **62.** Those at *greatest* risk for AIDS are
  (1) homosexual males
  (2) homosexual females
  (3) intravenous drug users
  (4) women whose sex partner is an active bisexual
  (5) heterosexuals with multiple sex partners
  A. All of these
  B. (1), (3), and (4)
  C. All except (1)
  D. (1) and (3)

_A_ **63.** AIDS is passed from one person to another through
  A. blood and body secretions
  B. sexual intercourse only
  C. drainage from open lesions only
  D. blood only

_D_ **64.** AIDS can be cured by
  A. sexual abstinence
  B. use of condoms
  C. single partner life-style
  D. none of these

_B_ **65.** When caring for the patient with AIDS, the nurse can help protect herself and others by
  (1) wearing gloves
  (2) frequent, careful handwashing
  (3) using special drainage and secretions precautions
  (4) recording fluid intake and output
  (5) administering anti-viral medications
  A. All of these
  B. (1), (2), and (3)
  C. (2), (4), and (5)
  D. (1), (3), and (5)

II. In the space before the treatment prescribed for patients with preeclampsia in Column I, place the letter of the rationale for the treatment from Column II.

	I TREATMENT PRESCRIBED		II RATIONALE FOR TREATMENT
_E_	**1.** Complete bed rest	**A.**	Indicates the response to treatment
_D_	**2.** Weigh daily	**B.**	Aids in determining efficiency of kidneys
_B_	**3.** Record fluid intake and output	**C.**	Relieves edema
_A_	**4.** Take blood pressure every 4 hours	**D.**	Indicates amount of fluids being eliminated from tissues
_A_	**5.** Check urine daily for albumin	**E.**	Slows metabolism
_F_	**6.** Sedatives	**F.**	Lowers blood pressure
_F_	**7.** Antihypertensive drugs		
_C_	**8.** Diuretics		

I.
1. C
2. B
3. D
4. A
5. C
6. D
7. B
8. A
9. D
10. C
11. A
12. C
13. B
14. D
15. D
16. C
17. B

18. A
19. C
20. A
21. C
22. A
23. B
24. B
25. A
26. D
27. B
28. D
29. B
30. D
31. B
32. C
33. D

34. B
35. A
36. D
37. C
38. D
39. A
40. B
41. D
42. B
43. C
44. A
45. D
46. B
47. C
48. A
49. B

50. B
51. D
52. B
53. C
54. B
55. C
56. A
57. C
58. B
59. B
60. C
61. B
62. D
63. A
64. D
65. B

II.
1. E
2. D
3. B

4. A
5. A
6. F

7. F
8. C

high-risk parents 17 and infants

I. SITUATION: While working in Dr. C.'s office this morning you took care of several expectant mothers:

Mrs. W., a 36-year-old gravida III, para I, who is in her eighth month of pregnancy. Her second pregnancy ended in a spontaneous abortion at 2½ months. Her other child was delivered by cesarean section because her pelvis is too small for vaginal deliveries. Her husband is an attorney; she is not employed outside the home.

Mrs. P., a 44-year-old gravida III, para II, who is seeing the doctor for the first time with this pregnancy. She has two grown daughters by a previous marriage. This will be her present husband's first child. Mrs. P. manages a restaurant; her husband is also a restaurant manager.

Mrs. A., a 30-year-old gravida III, para II, who had normal, spontaneous vaginal deliveries with her previous pregnancies. She is in her fourth month. Mrs. A. is a housewife; her husband is a mechanic.

Mrs. S., a 30-year-old gravida III, para I (she had one legal abortion). She is in her seventh month. She is Rh-negative. Mrs. S. is a clerk at a grocery store; her husband is a carpenter.

Karen, a 15-year-old unmarried gravida I, para 0, who is in her seventh month. She lives at home with her parents and two younger sisters. Her father is a truck driver and her mother is a waitress.

Mrs. O., a 22-year-old RN, who is a gravida I, para 0 in her eighth month of pregnancy. She is employed at the local hospital; her husband is a policeman.

Place the letter of the *best* answer in the space before the statement.

_____ **1.** Mrs. W. is likely to be considered high risk because of
- **A.** her age
- **B.** her socioeconomic status
- **C.** disease conditions
- **D.** problem pregnancies

_____ **2.** Mrs. P. may be considered high risk because of
- **(1)** her age
- **(2)** her marital status
- **(3)** disease conditions
- **(4)** problem pregnancies
- **A.** (1) only
- **B.** (2) and (3)
- **C.** (4) only
- **D.** None of these

_____ **3.** Mrs. A. may be considered high risk because of
- **(1)** her age
- **(2)** her parity
- **(3)** her socioeconomic status
- **(4)** problem pregnancies
- **A.** (1) and (2)
- **B.** (3) and (4)
- **C.** None of these
- **D.** All of these

_C_ **4.** Mrs. S. may be considered high risk because of
   (1) her age
   (2) her socioeconomic status
   (3) problem pregnancies
   (4) her parity
   A. (1) and (3)
   B. (2) and (4)
   C. (3) only
   D. None of these

_B_ **5.** Karen may be considered high risk because of
   (1) her age
   (2) disease conditions
   (3) her marital status
   (4) her parity
   A. All of these
   B. (1) and (3)
   C. (2) and (4)
   D. None of these

_A_ **6.** Mrs. O. may be considered high risk because of
   (1) her age
   (2) her socioeconomic status
   (3) disease conditions
   (4) problem pregnancies
   A. None of these
   B. All of these
   C. All except (1)
   D. (2) only

_D_ **7.** During Mrs. P.'s visit with the doctor, he discussed with her the problems commonly encountered when women her age become pregnant. Problems associated with pregnancy in women of Mrs. P.'s age include
   (1) higher maternal mortality
   (2) increased perinatal mortality
   (3) increased incidence of genetic abnormalities
   (4) increased incidence of chronic hypertensive vascular disease
   A. (1) and (2)
   B. (3) only
   C. (3) and (4)
   D. All of these

_A_ **8.** The problem most likely to develop with Mrs. S.'s pregnancy is
   A. Rh incompatibility
   B. anemia
   C. diabetes
   D. preeclampsia

_C_ **9.** In addition to caring for Mrs. S., the doctor probably will want Mr. S. checked for
   A. hemoglobin and hematocrit
   B. blood sugar
   C. Rh factor
   D. blood pressure

_C_ **10.** The only way the problem in question 8 would develop is if
   A. Mrs. S.'s hemoglobin is over 12.5 and her hematocrit is over 35.
   B. Mrs. S.'s blood sugar is over 100 mg/dl
   C. Mr. S. is Rh-positive and the fetus is Rh-positive
   D. Mrs. S.'s blood pressure is below 140/90

_D_ **11.** Dr. C. wants to know if Mrs. S. is producing antibodies against Rh-positive blood cells. The test he ordered for this is
   A. Rho (D) immune globulin
   B. kernicterus
   C. intrauterine transfusion
   D. antibody titer

_B_ **12.** Even though the conditions for Rh incompatibility were present with her other pregnancies and are present with this one, it probably will not develop
    A. since an antibody titer was done on Mrs. S.
    B. if Mrs. S. received Rho (D) immune globulin after both of her previous pregnancies
    C. if Mrs. S. received Rho (D) immune globulin after her first pregnancy
    D. if this fetus is given an intrauterine transfusion

_A_ **13.** The problems associated with pregnancies in women of Karen's age include
    (1) higher maternal mortality
    (2) increased perinatal mortality
    (3) preeclampsia
    (4) diabetes
    A. (1), (2), and (3)
    B. (2), (3), and (4)
    C. (1), (2), and (4)
    D. All of these

_A_ **14.** One reason Karen is considered high risk is because of her marital status. Which of the following is *not* true regarding unmarried mothers?
    A. they receive more antepartal care than married mothers
    B. they have more complications of pregnancy
    C. they have a higher rate of premature births and thus a greater risk of neonatal death
    D. they usually receive antepartal care at clinics and hospitals rather than from private physicians

_D_ **15.** During this visit, Dr. C. asked you to do a "roll-over" test on Karen. If this test is positive, it would mean Karen should be
    A. treated for syphilis
    B. treated for gonorrhea
    C. treated for diabetes
    D. watched closely for symptoms of preeclampsia

_A_ **16.** Since Karen has learned to trust you, she wishes to discuss with you what she should do with the baby when it is born. Probably the best thing you can do is to
    A. listen while she tells you how she feels about keeping or giving up the baby
    B. tell her she should keep the baby
    C. tell her she should give the baby up for adoption
    D. tell her to let her parents decide what should be done

_D_ **17.** The only complaint Mrs. O. had at this visit was swelling of her feet and ankles at the end of the day. You probably would
    (1) consider this a sign of preeclampsia
    (2) explain this is normal at this stage of pregnancy
    (3) find out if it disappears after a night's rest
    (4) suggest that she quit working until after the baby comes
    A. (1) only
    B. (1) and (4)
    C. (2) only
    D. (2) and (3)

_C_ **18.** Effects a high-risk condition may have on an expectant mother and/or her family may include
    (1) disruption of home routines
    (2) restriction of the mother's activities
    (3) decrease in stress
    (4) inability of the mother to complete the developmental tasks of pregnancy
    (5) strained relationships
    (6) lack of bonding with the infant
    A. All of these
    B. (1), (3), and (6)
    C. All except (3)
    D. (2), (4), and (5)

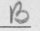

19. Nursing interventions for high-risk patients and their families might include
(1) helping them obtain correct, appropriate information
(2) reinforcing what the physician tells them
(3) being realistic about the possible outcome of the pregnancy
(4) helping them to accept the pregnancy as real and to develop emotional attachments to the infant
(5) encouraging them to discuss their feelings and fantasies about the infant
A. All except (5)
B. All of these
C. (1), (4), and (5)
D. (2), (3), and (4)

II. PROJECTS
1. Go through the file of prenatal records sent in by the physicians who practice obstetrics at your hospital and pick out the patients that you would consider high risk for each of the following reasons. List how their care might differ from that of normal-risk patients.

A. Age

B. Socioeconomic status

C. Marital status

D. Disease conditions

E. Problem pregnancies

F. Parity

G. Other conditions

2. Find out if your hospital has a newborn intensive care unit. If so, list the types of conditions most commonly found among the infants treated in it. If not, find out where the nearest Level III hospital (a hospital with a newborn intensive care unit) is located. Are any high-risk infants cared for at your hospital?

I.
1. D
2. A
3. C
4. C
5. B

6. A
7. D
8. A
9. C
10. C

11. D
12. B
13. A
14. A
15. D

16. A
17. D
18. C
19. B

variations of normal 18 labor and delivery

I. SITUATION: Linda and Dave arrived at the hospital labor suite at 1:15 A.M. They had gone to bed at 11:30 P.M. and at 12:30 A.M. Linda's membranes ruptured. Dave called the doctor and he told him to take her to the hospital even though she was not in labor yet. This is their first pregnancy.

After Linda was admitted Dave went home. At 3:30 A.M. Linda phoned him to let him know her labor had started. He returned to the hospital. By 5 P.M. Linda was completely dilated. After she had pushed for an hour the baby's head could be seen when the vulva was separated. The doctor then decided that he would deliver the baby with forceps. Linda was taken to the delivery room where, after she was prepped, the doctor gave her a pudendal block, did an L.M.L. episiotomy, and delivered the baby with Tucker-McLean forceps.

Place the letter of the *best* answer in the space before the statement.

_C_ **1.** The type of delivery Linda had would be called
  A. spontaneous
  B. midforceps
  C. low, or outlet, forceps
  D. high forceps

_A_ **2.** Tucker-McLean forceps have
  A. smooth, solid blades
  B. separated shanks
  C. fenestrated blades
  D. extra long, curved shanks

_B_ **3.** Forceps are used to
  (1) apply traction on the baby's head
  (2) apply traction on the baby's buttocks
  (3) rotate the baby's buttocks
  (4) rotate the baby's head
  A. All of these
  B. (1) and (4)
  C. (1) and (3)
  D. (2) and (3)

Mrs. W. is a gravida III, para I whose estimated date of confinement is March 25. Her first baby was delivered by cesarean section because of cephalopelvic disproportion (CPD). Her second pregnancy ended in spontaneous abortion at 2½ months gestation. She is scheduled for cesarean section on March 18.

_B_ **4.** The reason Mrs. W. is having a cesarean section this time is because of
  A. CPD
  B. previous cesarean section
  C. placenta previa
  D. fetal distress

_D_ **5.** If Mrs. W. has her cesarean section on March 18 as scheduled, the length of the gestation will be
  A. 42 weeks
  B. 40 weeks
  C. 41 weeks
  D. 39 weeks

_C_ **6.** The preoperative care Mrs. W. receives will
   (1) be the same as for anyone having abdominal surgery
   (2) include a retention catheter in the bladder
   (3) include listening to the fetal heart tones prior to surgery
   (4) include the same medication as for anyone having abdominal surgery
   A. All of these
   B. (1) and (4)
   C. (1), (2), and (3)
   D. (2), (3), and (4)

_B_ **7.** The problems that may be associated with spinal anesthesia include
   (1) aspiration of vomitus by the patient while anesthetized
   (2) maternal hypotension
   (3) severe postoperative headaches
   (4) maternal hypertension
   A. (1) and (4)
   B. (2) and (3)
   C. (1) and (2)
   D. (3) and (4)

_A_ **8.** The problems that may be associated with general anesthesia when used for cesarean section include
   (1) aspiration of vomitus by the patient while anesthetized
   (2) respiratory depression in the infant at birth
   (3) maternal hypotension
   (4) severe postoperative headaches
   A. (1) and (2)
   B. (3) and (4)
   C. (2) and (3)
   D. All of these

_B_ **9.** Measures that are taken to reduce the risk of respiratory depression in the infant when general anesthesia is used for cesarean section include
   A. elevation of the mother's legs
   B. prepping and draping the mother before the anesthetic is given
   C. using the left lateral recumbent position during transport to the operating room
   D. administering oxygen and intravenous glucose

_A_ **10.** The delivery nurse's responsibilities during a cesarean section consist of
   (1) assisting the pediatrician
   (2) having a heated crib or incubator ready for the baby
   (3) having oxygen and resuscitative equipment ready
   (4) identifying the infant and instilling the eye medication
   A. All of these
   B. (1) and (4)
   C. (2) and (3)
   D. (2) and (4)

Mrs. F. is a gravida III, para II whose estimated date of confinement is April 10. Her husband is a mining engineer. They live about 35 miles from the hospital where she plans to give birth. She had a 4-hour labor with her first baby, and a 2-hour labor with her second. In discussing her fears of giving birth before reaching the hospital, she and her doctor decided that, when the baby was mature enough and her cervix was favorable, he would induce labor. During her visit to his office 2 weeks before her due date, the doctor examined Mrs. F. and found that her cervix was 3 cm dilated and completely effaced. He ordered an ultrasound scanning (see Chap. 9) to find out the fetal age and size. The ultrasound report indicated that the baby was at 38 weeks' gestation and weighed 7¼ lb (3,289 g). The doctor requested that Mrs. F. be admitted to the hospital; he would begin the induction of labor as soon as his office closed at 5:30 P.M. In the meantime, a phone call was made to Mr. F. at his job so that he could be at the hospital by the time the induction was begun.

When Mrs. F. arrived at the hospital, she was given a partial shave but no enema. The fetal monitor was attached to Mrs. F.'s abdomen and an intravenous infusion of 1,000 ml of 5% glucose in water was started. Mr. F. and the doctor arrived at 6 P.M. At 6:10 P.M., 1,000 ml of 5% glucose in water containing five units of oxytocin was connected to the infusion pump and then added piggyback to the first I.V. The rate was set at 24 ml/hour. By 6:40 P.M., Mrs. F. was having contractions 3 to 4 minutes apart and lasting 30 to 45 seconds. The doctor then did an amniotomy. She was 4 to 5 cm dilated. At 7:15 P.M. Mrs. F. gave birth to a 7 lb 6 oz (3,345 g) baby boy who cried lustily and appeared normal in every way.

_D_ **11.** The reason for Mrs. F.'s induction was for
    A. obstetrical problems
    B. the doctor's convenience
    C. medical problems
    D. her convenience

_A_ **12.** From Mrs. F.'s experience you would understand a favorable cervix for induction to be one that is
    A. thin and partially dilated
    B. thin and undilated
    C. thick and partially dilated
    D. thick and undilated

_D_ **13.** By using the "piggyback" method when inducing labor,
    (1) the nurse is alerted when the I.V. tubing is occluded
    (2) the nurse is alerted when there is air in the tubing
    (3) the rate of flow is precisely controlled
    (4) the oxytocin infusion can be temporarily or permanently discontinued while the I.V. is still maintained
    A. All of these
    B. All except (4)
    C. (3) and (4)
    D. (4) only

_B_ **14.** By using an infusion pump when inducing labor,
    (1) the nurse is alerted when the I.V. tubing is occluded
    (2) the nurse is alerted when there is air in the tubing
    (3) the rate of flow is precisely controlled
    (4) the oxytocin infusion can be temporarily or permanently discontinued while the I.V. is maintained
    A. All of these
    B. All except (4)
    C. (3) and (4)
    D. (4) only

_C_ **15.** You would have decreased or discontinued the oxytocin infusion if
    (1) Mrs. F.'s contractions lasted 70 seconds
    (2) Mrs. F.'s contractions lasted 2 minutes
    (3) Mrs. F.'s blood pressure became elevated and remained elevated between contractions
    (4) the fetal heart rate slowed to 90 at the peak of each contraction and did not return to normal within 10 to 15 seconds after the contraction ended
    A. All of these
    B. (4) only
    C. All except (1)
    D. (3) and (4)

Mrs. C. is a gravida II, para I who had a 12-hour labor with her first baby. She was admitted to the hospital at 2:30 A.M. with good quality contractions 3 minutes apart and lasting 40 to 50 seconds. Her cervix was 80% effaced and 3 cm dilated. She stated that her labor had started about midnight. She continued to have good quality contractions at 3-minute intervals until 5 A.M., when they became weak and irregular. At that time she was 5 cm dilated. Although she was tired, she said she could not go to sleep because every time she tried, she would have a contraction.

_C_ **16.** The type of labor Mrs. C. experienced is called
    A. normal
    B. primary inertia
    C. hypotonic uterine dysfunction
    D. hypertonic uterine dysfunction

_B_ **17.** The treatment the doctor will order for Mrs. C. may include
    (1) a high, hot edema
    (2) sedation
    (3) x-ray pelvimetry
    (4) oxytocin infusion
    A. (1) and (4)
    B. (3) and (4)
    C. (1) and (2)
    D. (2) and (4)

_A_ **18.** If Mrs. C. complained of severe backache, you might suspect that
  A. the baby is in a posterior position
  B. the baby is in a breech position
  C. she has cephalopelvic disproportion
  D. she has supine hypotensive syndrome

_A_ **19.** If Mrs. C.'s baby is in a posterior position, you would understand that
  (1) the baby is looking up instead of down
  (2) if it rotates the backache will be relieved
  (3) it may be helpful for Mrs. C. to push on her side during second stage labor
  (4) Mrs. C. will appreciate backrubs during labor
  A. All of these
  B. All except (4)
  C. (1) and (2)
  D. (3) and (4)

_D_ **20.** Breech presentations occur in approximately
  A. 33% of all deliveries
  B. 30% of all deliveries
  C. 97% of all deliveries
  D. 3% of all deliveries

_D_ **21.** In a complete breech presentation
  A. one foot presents
  B. both feet present
  C. the buttocks present and the legs are extended up over the abdomen and chest
  D. the buttocks and feet present and the legs are flexed

_A_ **22.** Possible dangers associated with breech presentations include
  (1) hemorrhage
  (2) prolapsed cord
  (3) infection
  (4) head too large
  A. (2) and (4)
  B. (1) and (3)
  C. (1) and (2)
  D. (3) and (4)

_C_ **23.** Meconium in the amniotic fluid in a breech presentation is due to
  A. prolapsed cord
  B. fetal distress
  C. pressure on the buttocks
  D. molding of the fetal head

_A_ **24.** When cephalopelvic disproportion is present,
  (1) the baby's head is too large for the mother's pelvis
  (2) the mother's pelvis is too small for the baby's head
  (3) the baby's head does not descend even though dilatation occurs
  (4) the baby will probably be born by cesarean section
  A. All of these
  B. (1) and (2)
  C. (3) and (4)
  D. (1) and (4)

When you answered Mrs. C.'s call light, you found her lying in bed on her back. She said she felt light-headed and dizzy, like she was going to pass out.

_C_ **25.** You would
  A. suspect that she is hemorrhaging and notify the doctor
  B. suspect that her blood sugar is low and give her some sweetened orange juice
  C. suspect that she has supine hypotensive syndrome and position her on her side
  D. suspect that delivery is imminent and notify the doctor

II. PROJECTS

1. Compare the different types of obstetrical forceps commonly used and find out the difference between:

   A. Simpson forceps and Elliot forceps

   B. Tucker-McLean forceps and Luikart-Simpson (also called Luikart-McLean forceps)

2. Find out what the following forceps are used for:

   A. Piper forceps

   B. Keilland forceps

3. Interview a postoperative cesarean section patient and find out:

   A. Why she had a cesarean section

   B. How long beforehand she knew she was going to have a cesarean section

   C. How she felt when she found out she was going to have a cesarean section

   D. How she feels about having another cesarean section

   E. How her husband felt about their baby being born by cesarean section

III. In the space before the statement in Column I, place the letter of the step it describes in a nursing care plan, from Column II.

	I STATEMENT	II STEPS IN A NURSING CARE PLAN

_A_	1. Determine the progress of labor
_D_	2. Early detection of problems
_C_	✓3. Examine patient
_C_	4. Note frequency, duration, and intensity of contractions
_D_	5. Patient (couple) verbalizes understanding of labor complication
_B_	6. Potential for injury, lack of progress of labor related to baby's position or presentation, or cephalopelvic disproportion
_A_	7. Observe physical response of patient to prolonged labor
_B_	8. Knowledge deficit related to labor complication
_D_	9. Patient is as comfortable as possible
_C_	10. Explain apparent problem and the interventions being undertaken to correct it
_B_	11. Fluid volume deficit related to low fluid intake
_A_	✓12. Monitor intake and output
_C_	13. Give intravenous fluids as ordered
_D_	14. Receives fluids needed
_A_	15. Monitor fetal heart rate
_C_	16. Report abnormal fetal heart rate
_B_	17. Ineffective individual coping related to fatigue and discouragement because of prolonged labor
_C_	18. Listen to patient (couple)
_C_	19. Report meconium in amniotic fluid
_C_	20. Stay with patient (couple)
_A_	21. Observe psychological/emotional response of patient (couple) to prolonged labor
_D_	22. Birth is accomplished safely for mother and infant
_B_	23. Disturbance in self-concept related to inability to have method of childbirth desired
_D_	24. Able to accept the fact that she was not to blame
_B_	25. Fear related to safety of mother and infant
_C_	26. Reassure patient (couple)
_B_	27. Alteration in comfort: pain related to prolonged labor
_D_	28. Receives support she needs
_C_	29. Assist doctor with exams
_C_	30. Prepare for delivery: vaginal or cesarean section

A. Assessment
B. Potential Nursing Diagnosis
C. Intervention
D. Expected Outcome

I. **1.** C   **8.** A   **15.** C   **22.** A

2. A   **9.** B   **16.** C   **23.** C

3. B   **10.** A   **17.** B   **24.** A

4. B   **11.** D   **18.** A   **25.** C

5. D   **12.** A   **19.** A

6. C   **13.** D   **20.** D

7. B   **14.** B   **21.** D

II. **1.** **A.** The shanks are separated on Simpson forceps and together on Elliot forceps.

B. Tucker-McLean forceps have smooth solid blades; Luikart-Simpson forceps have a single ridge on solid blades.

2. **A.** Piper forceps are used to deliver the aftercoming head in breech delivery.

B. Keilland forceps are used to rotate the position of the baby's head.

III. **1.** A   **9.** D   **17.** B   **24.** D

2. D   **10.** C   **18.** C   **25.** B

3. C   **11.** B   **19.** C   **26.** C

4. C   **12.** A   **20.** C   **27.** B

5. D   **13.** C   **21.** A   **28.** D

6. B   **14.** D   **22.** D   **29.** C

7. A   **15.** A   **23.** B   **30.** C

8. B   **16.** C

problems during the puerperium 19

I. SITUATION: Mrs. G. is an attractive red-haired gravida II, para I who had a 6-hour labor with her first child, Jeffrey, who weighed 7 lb 15 oz (3,600 g). Today her labor started about 1:15 P.M. and, although she wasted no time getting her 2-year-old son to her friend's and calling her husband, she was 6 cm dilated by the time she arrived at the hospital at 2 P.M. At 2:20 P.M. her membranes ruptured spontaneously and at 2:26 P.M. she gave birth to an 8 lb 13 oz (3,997 g) boy. At 2:35 P.M., the placenta delivered spontaneously and appeared to be intact and complete. Her blood pressure was 120/70 and her pulse was 76. The doctor ordered Pitocin 10 units I.M. At 2:45 P.M., Mr. G. arrived and Mrs. G. informed him that he now has a second son. Mrs. G.'s doctor told the nurse that, if needed, she should start an intravenous infusion of 1,000 ml of 5% glucose in water and add 20 units of Pitocin to it.

Place the letter of the *best* answer in the space before the statement.

_A_   **1.** Mrs. G.'s labor probably would be most accurately classified as
     A. rapid
     B. long
     C. difficult
     D. desultory

_C_   **2.** The size of Mrs. G.'s second son probably would be best described as
     A. small
     B. average
     C. large
     D. below average

_B_   **3.** The reason the doctor ordered an oxytocin infusion, if needed, was because he thought Mrs. G. might have
     A. laceration of the perineum
     B. uterine atony
     C. retained placental fragments
     D. puerperal infection

_D_   **4.** You would give Mrs. G. the oxytocin infusion if you found that
     (1) the uterus was contracted and at her umbilicus
     (2) the uterus was boggy and two fingerbreadths above the umbilicus
     (3) the bleeding was moderate without clots
     (4) the bleeding was heavy with clots
     A. (1) and (3)
     B. (1) and (4)
     C. (2) and (3)
     D. (2) and (4)

_D_   **5.** You would consider that Mrs. G. had a postpartum hemorrhage if her blood loss was more than
     A. 200 ml
     B. 300 ml
     C. 400 ml
     D. 500 ml

B   6. If you found that Mrs. G.'s uterus was relaxed, the *first* thing you should do is to
  - **A.** notify the doctor
  - **B.** massage it until it is firm
  - **C.** press on it to empty it of blood and clots
  - **D.** start the oxytocin infusion

A   7. If Mrs. G. was bleeding too much although her uterus was firmly contracted, you would suspect the cause to be
  - **A.** lacerations of the cervix or birth canal
  - **B.** uterine atony
  - **C.** retained cotyledons
  - **D.** retained pieces of membranes

Mrs. S. is a 36-year-old mother of six whose youngest child was born 2 days ago. When you answer her call signal she tells you that she is having pain in her leg. You inspect the area and find that it is slightly swollen and reddened in appearance and feels cordlike when you touch it. Mrs. S. says it is very tender and painful when touched.

C   8. The *first* thing you should do after examining Mrs. S's leg is to
  - **A.** massage the leg to improve circulation
  - **B.** give her an analgesic
  - **C.** report your findings to her doctor
  - **D.** give her an oxytocic

A   9. When you notify the doctor, he confirms your suspicions that Mrs. S. probably has a form of puerperal infection called
  - **A.** thrombophlebitis
  - **B.** septicemia
  - **C.** endometritis
  - **D.** parametritis

B   10. Which of the following would the doctor never prescribe in the treatment of Mrs. S.?
  - **A.** elevate her feet and legs 30° to 45°
  - **B.** massage her affected leg
  - **C.** moist heat to the affected area
  - **D.** anticoagulants

D   11. The organism which causes most puerperal infections is
  - **A.** staphylococcus
  - **B.** colon bacillus
  - **C.** gonococcus
  - **D.** streptococcus

A   12. One of the most important measures that can be taken to prevent puerperal infection is
  - **A.** frequent and thorough handwashing
  - **B.** isolation of mothers with infection
  - **C.** maintaining strict asepsis in the delivery room
  - **D.** providing each mother with cleansed and autoclaved equipment

B   13. If the doctor prescribed anticoagulants for Mrs. S., you would observe her closely for signs of
  - **A.** spread of the infection
  - **B.** hemorrhage from the uterus
  - **C.** a dislodged thrombus
  - **D.** formation of additional thrombi

C   14. Mastitis is most commonly caused by
  - **A.** hemolytic streptococcus
  - **B.** beta streptococcus
  - **C.** *Staphylococcus aureus*
  - **D.** colon bacillus

A   15. The organism producing mastitis may be carried to the breasts
  - **(1)** by the infant when nursing
  - **(2)** on the hands of the mother
  - **(3)** on the hands of the nurse
  - **(4)** on the hands of the doctor
  - **A.** All of these
  - **B.** All except (1)
  - **C.** (3) and (4)
  - **D.** (3) only

_C_ **16.** The organism causing mastitis may enter the breast through
  A. the bloodstream of the mother
  B. contaminated food the mother eats
  C. cracks in the mother's nipple
  D. invasion of the reproductive tract

_D_ **17.** Symptoms a mother with mastitis would experience include
  (1) chills and fever
  (2) frequent, painful urination
  (3) chest pain and shortness of breath
  (4) the lobe of the breast is reddened, painful, and feels hard to the touch
  A. (4) only
  B. (3) and (4)
  C. All except (2)
  D. (1) and (4)

_B_ **18.** Cystitis is most likely to occur when
  (1) a mother does not wipe from front to back when cleansing the perineal area
  (2) a mother is unable to empty her bladder completely when she urinates
  (3) a mother's bladder is allowed to become overly distended
  (4) careful asepsis is not practiced during catheterization
  A. (1) only
  B. All except (1)
  C. (2) and (4)
  D. (3) and (4)

_A_ **19.** When checking for residual urine, catheterization should be done within
  A. 5 minutes after a voiding
  B. 10 minutes after a voiding
  C. 15 minutes after a voiding
  D. 25 minutes after a voiding

_B_ **20.** Residual urine is considered present if, on catheterization following a voiding, the amount of urine obtained is
  A. 30 ml or more
  B. 60 ml or more
  C. 90 ml or more
  D. 120 ml or more

_D_ **21.** The symptoms a mother with cystitis may experience include
  (1) chills and fever
  (2) frequent, painful urination
  (3) pain in her lower abdomen
  (4) a feeling of not having emptied her bladder
  A. (1) and (2)
  B. (2) and (4)
  C. All except (3)
  D. All of these

II. In the space before the term in Column I, place the letter of its definition from Column II.

I
TERM

II
DEFINITION

_E_ **1.** Cystitis

_C_ **2.** Endometritis

_H_ **3.** Mastitis

_G_ **4.** Parametritis

_A_ **5.** Puerperal infection

_D_ **6.** Puerperal morbidity

_F_ **7.** Septicemia

_B_ **8.** Thrombophlebitis

_I_ **9.** Pulmonary embolism

A. Invasion of the reproductive tract by pathogenic organisms

B. Inflammation of the pelvic or femoral veins

C. Infection of the lining of the uterus

D. A temperature of 100.4°F (38°C) or higher on 2 consecutive days during the first 10 days postpartum, excluding the first 24 hours

E. Inflammation of the bladder caused by bacteria

F. Generalized infection in which the organisms invade the bloodstream

G. Infection in the connective tissue around the uterus

H. Inflammation of the breasts

I. Occlusion of the pulmonary artery by a thrombus

III. In the space before the treatment for puerperal infection in Column I, place the letter of the purpose for the treatment from Column II.

I
TREATMENT PRESCRIBED

II
PURPOSE OF TREATMENT

_B_ **1.** Bed rest

_G_ **2.** Culture of drainage and/or blood

_E_ **3.** Force fluids

_I_ **4.** High-calorie, high-vitamin diet

_A_ **5.** Analgesics

_J_ **6.** Ergonovine maleate (Ergotrate) (endometritis)

_D_ **7.** Elevate head of bed (endometritis)

_H_ **8.** Elevate feet and legs (thrombophlebitis)

_F_ **9.** Moist or dry heat (thrombophlebitis)

_C_ **10.** Anticoagulants (thrombophlebitis)

A. Promote comfort

B. Conserve energy and provide rest

C. Prevent formation of additional thrombi

D. Promote drainage from uterus

E. Promote body functions

F. Help decrease size of thrombus

G. Determine most effective antibiotic or sulfonamide drug

H. Aid return circulation from feet and legs

I. Help build up resistance

J. Keep uterus contracted and thus prevent spread of infection to surrounding areas

IV. In the space before the potential nursing diagnosis, write **A** if it would be *most* appropriate for a patient with postpartum hemorrhage, **B** if it would be *most* appropriate for a patient with puerperal infection, or **C** if it would be equally appropriate for either.

POTENTIAL NURSING DIAGNOSIS

CONDITION

__C__ **1.** Knowledge deficit related to her condition

__A__ **2.** Alteration in comfort: pain related to massage of uterus

__B__ **3.** Anxiety related to her condition and her inability to care for infant

__A__ **4.** Potential for injury, hemorrhage related to relaxed uterus, retained placental fragments or lacerations of birth canal

__C__ **5.** Fear related to her well-being

__B__ **6.** Anxiety related to her condition and the added expense of prolonged hospitalization

__B__ **7.** Sleep pattern disturbance related to her illness

__A__ **8.** Fear related to AIDS if blood transfusions are necessary

A. Postpartum hemorrhage

B. Puerperal infection

C. Both

I.
1. A
2. C
3. B
4. D
5. D
6. B
7. A
8. C
9. A
10. B
11. D
12. A
13. B
14. C
15. A
16. C
17. D
18. B
19. A
20. B
21. D

II.
1. E
2. C
3. H
4. G
5. A
6. D
7. F
8. B
9. I

III.
1. B
2. G
3. E
4. I
5. A
6. J
7. D
8. H
9. F
10. C

IV.
1. C
2. A
3. B
4. A
5. C
6. B
7. B
8. A

problems of the 20 newborn

I. **SITUATION:** Baby R.'s mother was diagnosed as a diabetic about 2 years before she became pregnant for the first time. During the latter part of her pregnancy, Mrs. R. was treated for preeclampsia. Although Mrs. R.'s labor was relatively short, lasting less than 8 hours, delivery was complicated by shoulder dystocia. One minute after birth, Baby R.'s heart rate was 110, her respirations were slow and irregular, her color was blue, there was some flexion of her extremities, and she grimaced when she was suctioned with the catheter. Five minutes after birth her heart rate was 140, her respirations were good, there was some flexion of her extremities, and she cried when stimulated. However, she was given oxygen because her color was still blue.

The pediatrician was present for the birth and he decided that since the birth had been difficult for Baby R., he would take her to the nursery right away. In the nursery Baby R. was weighed before she was placed in an incubator and given oxygen. She weighed 8 lb 8 oz (3,856 g). A Dextrostix showed her blood sugar to be 35 mg. The pediatrician started an intravenous infusion, via her umbilical vein, of a 10% solution of glucose.

In addition to the observations made of normal newborns, Baby R. was observed closely for signs of problems common to infants of diabetic mothers. An x-ray film taken of her shoulder showed that no fracture was present.

Within a few hours after birth, Baby R.'s color was pink without the administered oxygen, and her muscle tone was good. Within 24 hours after birth she was taking and retaining her formula feedings well, so the pediatrician discontinued her IV. Her temperature was stable and, except for tenderness in her shoulder, she appeared to be in excellent condition. She was removed from the incubator and placed in a crib, although the close observation for possible problems was continued.

Place the letter of the *best* answer in the space before the statement.

____D____ **1.** At 1 minute after birth, you would give Baby R. an Apgar score of
    A. 10
    B. 7
    C. 9
    D. 5

____B____ **2.** At 5 minutes after birth, you would give her an Apgar score of
    A. 10
    B. 7
    C. 9
    D. 5

____C____ **3.** Baby R. probably would be considered
    A. postmature
    B. appropriate for gestational age
    C. large for gestational age
    D. small for gestational age

____A____ **4.** The excessive size of infants born to diabetic mothers is due to
    A. hyperglycemia in the mother and hyperinsulinism in the fetus
    B. hyperinsulinism in the mother and hyperglycemia in the fetus
    C. hyperinsulinism in the fetus and hypoglycemia in the mother
    D. hypoglycemia in the fetus and hyperinsulinism in the mother

_D_ 5. Because Baby R.'s system continues to produce large quantities of insulin even though she stopped receiving a large supply of glucose from her mother at birth, she must be observed closely for
   A. hyperbilirubinemia
   B. respiratory distress syndrome
   C. hypocalcemia
   D. hypoglycemia

_C_ 6. If Baby R. had not breathed within 30 to 60 seconds after birth, she would have had a condition known as
   A. respiratory distress syndrome
   B. narcosis
   C. asphyxia neonatorum
   D. anoxia

_C_ 7. Baby R. was observed closely for symptoms of respiratory distress syndrome. Which of the following would *not* be symptoms?
   A. grunty respirations accompanied by flaring of the nostrils and retraction of the chest wall
   B. seesaw breathing
   C. irregular, abdominal breathing
   D. rapid, labored breathing

_A_ 8. Respiratory distress syndrome is caused by
   (1) a hyaline membrane forming in the lining of the alveoli of the lungs resulting in atelectasis of that part of the lung
   (2) bacteria entering the uterus during a prolonged labor or following early rupture of the membranes
   (3) the infant aspirating fluid during birth or following a feeding
   (4) bacteria and viruses coming in contact with the infant in the nursery
   A. (1) only
   B. All except (1)
   C. (2) and (4)
   D. All of these

_B_ 9. The treatment of respiratory distress syndrome includes
   A. antibiotics
   B. incubator and oxygen
   C. phototherapy
   D. exchange transfusions

_D_ 10. Other problems which may develop in infants of Baby R.'s size and gestational age include
   (1) hyperbilirubinemia
   (2) hypocalcemia
   (3) phocomelia
   (4) phenylketonuria
   A. All of these
   B. (3) and (4)
   C. (2) and (3)
   D. (1) and (2)

_D_ 11. Parents' reactions, when told that their newborn infant has a problem, may be influenced by
   (1) when and how they are told
   (2) the seriousness of the problem and whether or not it can be corrected
   (3) whether it may recur with future pregnancies
   (4) their emotional and spiritual maturity
   A. (1) and (4)
   B. (2) and (3)
   C. (2), (3), and (4)
   D. All of these

B 12. In her contacts with parents of infants with problems, the nurse should
   (1) realize that parents may react in various ways when informed that their infant has a problem
   (2) spare the parents anxiety by delaying telling them their infant has a problem
   (3) tell them of other families she's known who have had the same, or similar, problems
   (4) be able to provide support to the parents and to answer their questions intelligently
   A. All of these
   B. (1) and (4)
   C. (2) and (3)
   D. All except (3)

A 13. The developmental defect which causes more deaths during the first year of life than any other defect is
   A. congenital heart defects
   B. cleft lip and cleft palate
   C. phocomelia
   D. spina bifida

C 14. A major problem encountered when caring for infants who have a cleft lip or a cleft palate is
   A. the excessive size of the head
   B. infection
   C. feeding
   D. paralysis of the trunk and lower extremities

A 15. The care of an infant with a cleft lip or a cleft palate includes
   (1) frequent suctioning
   (2) keeping the lips moist with an ointment or oil
   (3) holding the infant in an upright position to feed and burping the infant frequently
   (4) teaching the mother to feed the infant
   A. All of these
   B. All except (1)
   C. (3) and (4)
   D. (3) only

D 16. Which of the following conditions is *most* likely to cause a long labor and difficult delivery?
   A. spina bifida
   B. Down's syndrome
   C. phocomelia
   D. hydrocephalus

B 17. A drug-induced condition in which the infant is born without arms and/or legs or with stumps where the limbs should be is
   A. spina bifida
   B. phocomelia
   C. Down's syndrome
   D. hydrocephalus

A 18. A major problem encountered in caring for the hydrocephalic infant is
   A. the weight of the head
   B. infections
   C. paralysis of the bowel and bladder sphincters
   D. mental retardation

C 19. When performing passive overcorrection of the foot on an infant with clubfoot, you would
   A. observe the infant's toes and thighs for signs of circulatory impairment
   B. keep the knee flexed while holding the foot in a position as near to normal as possible for 5 minutes
   C. support the leg under the calf and flex the knee while pulling the entire foot as far as possible in the opposite direction and hold for 1 minute
   D. support the leg under the thigh and extend the knee while pulling the foot as far as possible in the opposite direction and hold for 1 minute

_D_ 20. The condition in which the infant has slanting eyes close together, a small head, thick neck, large protruding tongue, short, thick hands with simian creases across the palmar surfaces, and relaxed joints is
A. spina bifida
B. Rh incompatibility
C. phenylketonuria
D. Down's syndrome

_A_ 21. The most common cause of Down's syndrome is
A. trisomy 21
B. chromosomal translocation
C. chromosomal mosaicism
D. trisomy 15

_C_ 22. The treatment for phenylketonuria consists of
A. surgery
B. antibiotics
C. a special diet containing limited amounts of phenylalanine
D. phototherapy

_B_ 23. Tests that are performed on the cord blood of babies born to Rh-negative mothers include
(1) blood type and Rh
(2) hemoglobin and hematocrit
(3) serology and blood sugar
(4) Coombs and bilirubin
A. All of these
B. All except (3)
C. (1) and (4)
D. (2) and (3)

_A_ 24. Jaundice due to Rh incompatibility usually appears
A. within a few hours or a day or two after birth
B. on the third or fourth day of life
C. on the fifth or sixth day of life
D. within 2 weeks after birth

_D_ 25. ABO incompatibility can occur when the mother's blood type is
A. A and the baby's is O or B
B. B and the baby's is A or O
C. A or B and the baby's is O
D. O and the baby's is A or B

_B_ 26. The purpose of phototherapy is to
A. replace red blood cells
B. reduce bilirubin levels in the blood
C. destroy antibodies in the blood
D. increase the oxygen content of the blood

_D_ 27. Measures you should take when caring for an infant receiving phototherapy include
(1) uncovering the infant except for the diaper
(2) closing the eyes before covering them, then keeping them covered
(3) changing the infant's position periodically
(4) taking the infant's temperature and giving fluids at regular intervals
A. (2) only
B. (1) and (2)
C. All except (4)
D. All of these

_C_ 28. If you discovered an infant in the nursery with yellow, blisterlike lesions in the creases of the neck, arms, and thighs, you would suspect
A. thrush
B. drug addiction
C. impetigo
D. kernicterus

_A_ **29.** Examples of staphylococal infections which would occur in the nursery include
  (1) epidemic diarrhea
  (2) cord infections
  (3) thrush
  (4) impetigo
  A. (2) and (4)
  B. (1) only
  C. (2) and (3)
  D. (4) only

_B_ **30.** If you found white, curdlike patches resembling milk in the mouth of a newborn infant and they left a raw, bleeding area when you tried to wipe them off, you would suspect that the infant had
  A. impetigo
  B. thrush
  C. staphylococcal infection
  D. drug addiction

_C_ **31.** Symptoms which an infant with drug addiction might manifest include
  (1) restlessness and tremors
  (2) shrill cry and convulsions
  (3) twitchings of the extremities and/or face
  (4) yawning, sneezing, and excessive mucus
  A. (2) and (3)
  B. (1) and (3)
  C. All of these
  D. All except (4)

_A_ **32.** It is possible to detect hearing problems in infants as early as
  A. a day or two after birth
  B. a week or two after birth
  C. a month after birth
  D. 6 months after birth

II. In the space before the statement, write a **T** if the statement is true, or an **F** if it is false.

_F_ **1.** All parents who have a child who is less than normal eventually adapt to it.

_T_ **2.** The mental health, marriage, and relationship to the child of parents with an abnormal child are in jeopardy if they don't adapt.

_T_ **3.** A higher divorce rate and an increase in child abuse are found among parents of premature or sick infants.

_F_ **4.** Support groups are ineffective in helping parents of sick infants cope.

_T_ **5.** Parents who are able to cope find that their lives are permanently affected by the birth of a severely ill or anomalous infant who survives.

III. In the space before the type of nursing care plan in Column I, place the letter or letters of an appropriate potential nursing diagnosis from Column II.

I
NURSING CARE PLAN

_____ **1.** Grieving family

_____ **2.** Infant with respiratory distress syndrome

_____ **3.** Infant with jaundice due to Rh or ABO incompatibility

_____ **4.** Infant with infection

_____ **5.** Infant of a diabetic mother

II
POTENTIAL NURSING DIAGNOSIS

A. Potential for injury, kernicterus related to elevated bilirubin levels

B. Potential for infection related to immature immune system, environmental factors, exposure to maternal infection, or exposure to infection in nursery

C. Anticipatory or dysfunctional grieving

D. Impaired gas exchange related to lack of lung surfactant

E. Potential for injury at birth related to excessive size

F. Ineffective airway clearance related to increased secretions and decreased ability to cough

G. Knowledge deficit related to cause of death, anomaly, or illness; prognosis for sick infant; or probability for recurrence in future pregnancy

H. Potential for injury, dehydraton, conjunctivitis, or hyperthermia related to phototherapy

I. Potential fluid volume deficit and electrolyte imbalance

J. Ineffective individual or family coping

IV. In the space before the term in Column I, place the letter of its definition from Column II.

I
TERM

D **1.** Anoxia

K **2.** Asphyxia neonatorum

Q **3.** Atelectasis

H **4.** *Candida albicans*

V **5.** Cleft lip

R **6.** Cleft palate

M **7.** Clubfoot

B **8.** Down's syndrome

F **9.** *Escherichia coli*

O **10.** Hydrocephalus

P **11.** Kernicterus

T **12.** LSD-25

U **13.** Meningocele

W **14.** Myelomeningocele

L **15.** Narcosis

C **16.** Patent ductus arteriosus

S **17.** Patent foramen ovale

I **18.** Phocomelia

G **19.** Phototherapy

II
DEFINITION

A. A hereditary problem in which the body is unable to metabolize the protein phenylalanine

B. A disorder caused by chromosomal abnormalities, in which the infant has physical defects and mental retardation

C. A congenital heart defect in which the opening between the aorta and the pulmonary artery does not close after birth

D. Interference with the oxygen supply

E. An organism that may cause infections of the skin and umbilical areas of the newborn

F. One of the most dangerous organisms to the newborn, frequently the cause of epidemic diarrhea

G. Treatment by exposure to light

H. The organism that causes thrush in newborns

I. A drug-induced condition in which the infant is born without arms and/or legs or with stumps where the limbs should be

J. A lung infection which causes about 10% of newborn deaths

A 20. PKU

J 21. Pneumonia

X 22. Pyloric stenosis

N 23. Spina bifida

E 24. Staphylococcus

Y 25. Tracheoesophageal fistula

K. A condition in which the infant does not breathe for 30 to 60 seconds after birth

L. Respiratory depression in the newborn at birth as a result of analgesia and anesthesia given to the mother before delivery

M. A deformity in which there is an abnormal turning of one or both feet

N. A defect of the spine in which the bony part of the spinal canal fails to close

O. A condition in which an excessive amount of cerebrospinal fluid is generated in the ventricles of the brain

P. Severe, permanent brain damage caused by accumulation of large amounts of bilirubin in the brain

Q. Collapsed lung

R. A separation down the middle of the roof of the mouth

S. A congenital heart defect in which the opening between the right and left auricles of the heart does not close after birth

T. The drug, lysergic acid, that may cause an infant to be born with chromosomal abnormalities if the mother takes it before and during pregnancy

U. A condition in which the membranes of the spinal cord bulge through the opening in the spinal canal and form a soft sac filled with cerebrospinal fluid

V. A separation of the upper lip on one or both sides of the midline

W. A condition in which the nerve fibers as well as the membranes of the spinal cord protrude through the opening of the spinal canal in spina bifida

X. Narrowing of the lower opening of the stomach

Y. A tubelike passage between the esophagus and the trachea

I.
1. D
2. B
3. C
4. A
5. D
6. C
7. C
8. A
9. B
10. D
11. D
12. B
13. A
14. C
15. A
16. D
17. B
18. A
19. C
20. D
21. A
22. C
23. B
24. A
25. D
26. B
27. D
28. C
29. A
30. B
31. C
32. A

II.
1. F
2. T
3. T
4. F
5. T

III.
1. C, G, J
2. D, F, I
3. A, H, I
4. B, I
5. E, I

IV.
1. D
2. K
3. Q
4. H
5. V
6. R
7. M
8. B
9. F
10. O
11. P
12. T
13. U
14. W
15. L
16. C
17. S
18. I
19. G
20. A
21. J
22. X
23. N
24. E
25. Y

low birth weight and 21 preterm infants

I. **SITUATION:** Mr. and Mrs. S. have a daughter 5 years old and a son 2 years old. Another pregnancy ended in a spontaneous abortion at 2 months. Both parents are heavy smokers. Mrs. S.'s estimated date of confinement for this pregnancy was July 13. However, at 10 P.M. on May 30, she went into labor and at 12:46 A.M. on May 31, she gave birth to a 2 lb 12 oz (1,247 g) baby boy. During labor, Mrs. S. was coached in breathing methods to help her relax. She was cooperative when she understood why the doctor did not want her to have medication for pain.

The delivery nurse had alerted the intensive care nursery of the impending premature birth and had the resuscitation supplies ready before Mrs. S. was taken to the delivery room.

The pediatrician was present for the birth. As soon as the baby was born, the obstetrician cleared his airway, clamped his cord, and placed him in the heated crib. Very gently the nurse wiped him dry and the pediatrician listened to his heart and lungs and gently suctioned him. At birth, Baby S. cried spontaneously, his heart rate was 150, his color was pink, and he was active. Five minutes later he was less vigorous and his respirations were grunty. In the intensive care nursery an intravenous infusion was started and he was placed in an incubator with oxygen. His chest was x-rayed, and blood was drawn for laboratory tests. The pediatrician and nurse were with Baby S. constantly.

Place the letter of the *best* answer in the space before the statement.

_B_ 1. In addition to being premature, Baby S. would also be considered
(1) preterm
(2) AGA
(3) SGA
(4) LGA
A. (1) and (2)
B. (1) and (3)
C. (1) and (4)
D. (1) only

_C_ 2. Which of the following would be *least* likely to describe Baby S.?
A. round head, small face, large, bulging eyes
B. red, wrinkled, delicate, thin skin
C. elongated head, plump appearance
D. lanugo on face, arms, and back

_A_ 3. Of the many factors which may be responsible for growth retardation, the one which may have affected Baby S. is
A. heavy smoking by his mother
B. malnutrition
C. multiple pregnancy
D. genetic factors

_B_ 4. Medications that might have been used to try to stop Mrs. S.'s labor include
A. atropine or scopolamine
B. magnesium sulfate or ritodrine hydrochloride
C. calcium gluconate or phenothiazines
D. meperidine or diazepam

A   **5.** An increase in maternal and infant heart rates, an elevation in systolic and a decrease in diastolic maternal blood pressure, nausea, vomiting, tremors, headache, erythema, nervousness, jitteriness, and anxiety are symptoms you would look for when a woman in preterm labor is given
     A. ritodrine hydrochloride
     B. magnesium sulfate
     C. calcium gluconate
     D. meperidine

B   **6.** Depressed or absent reflexes, respirations less than 16 per minute, a urinary output less than 100 ml per 4 hours, excessive thirst, hot feelings, flaccid paralysis, circulatory collapse, or depressed cardiac function are symptoms you would look for when a woman in preterm labor is given
     A. ritodrine hydrochloride
     B. magnesium sulfate
     C. calcium gluconate
     D. meperidine

D   **7.** Problems to which Baby S. is highly susceptible because of his gestational age include
     (1) hypothermia
     (2) anemia
     (3) hypoglycemia
     (4) respiratory distress syndrome
     A. (1) and (4)
     B. (2) and (3)
     C. (4) only
     D. All of these

C   **8.** Problems to which Baby S. is highly susceptible because of his size include
     (1) congenital malformations
     (2) intrauterine infections
     (3) hypoglycemia
     (4) meconium aspiration
     A. (1) and (3)
     B. (2) and (4)
     C. All except (4)
     D. All of these

A   **9.** The reason Mrs. S. was not given medication for pain during labor was
     A. to lessen the chance of respiratory depression in the infant at birth
     B. to avoid the possibility of slowing or stopping her labor
     C. to punish her for going into labor prematurely
     D. so that she could be awake and actively participate in the birth

D   **10.** The grunty respirations which Baby S. developed soon after birth most likely are
     A. normal for an infant his size
     B. due to aspiration of mucus
     C. a symptom of pneumonia
     D. a symptom of respiratory distress syndrome

B   **11.** The leading cause of death among newborn infants in this country is
     A. postmaturity
     B. prematurity
     C. malformations
     D. respiratory distress syndrome

A   **12.** The most common cause of death among premature infants is
     A. respiratory distress syndrome
     B. infections
     C. birth injuries
     D. hypoglycemia

D   **13.** The purposes accomplished by putting Baby S. in an incubator include
     (1) maintaining a stable, desirable temperature
     (2) preventing infection by isolating him
     (3) making observation of him easy
     (4) making oxygen administration easy
     A. (1) only
     B. (4) only
     C. All except (3)
     D. All of these

_C_ **14.** The reasons for minimal and gentle handling of Baby S. are to
   (1) avoid injury to his fragile blood vessels with resultant hemorrhage into his tissues
   (2) promote his emotional well-being
   (3) conserve his limited supply of energy
   (4) prevent infection by avoiding injury to his tissues
   A. (1) and (3)
   B. (1) and (4)
   C. All except (2)
   D. All of these

_A_ **15.** Baby S.'s nervous system is immature. Consequently, oral feeding may be a problem because of the absence of certain reflexes, including
   (1) grasp
   (2) sucking
   (3) swallowing
   (4) Moro
   A. (2) and (3)
   B. (1) and (4)
   C. All except (4)
   D. All of these

_B_ **16.** Due to his immaturity and the absence of these reflexes, during the first days or week of life Baby S. probably will be fed by
   A. bottle
   B. intravenous infusion
   C. gavage
   D. breast

_D_ **17.** When oral feedings are started, you find that Baby S. regurgitates easily. This is most likely because
   (1) his stomach is narrow and upright
   (2) he dislikes the taste of the feeding
   (3) his stomach sphincters are poorly developed
   (4) he is overfed
   A. (1) only
   B. (2) and (4)
   C. (3) only
   D. (1) and (3)

_B_ **18.** Unless Baby S.'s color and respirations indicate that higher concentrations of oxygen are necessary, it would be best to keep the concentration of oxygen below
   A. 20%
   B. 40%
   C. 60%
   D. 80%

_A_ **19.** Controlling the oxygen concentration Baby S. receives is done to prevent
   A. retrolental fibroplasia
   B. ophthalmia neonatorum
   C. purpura
   D. hyperbilirubinemia

_D_ **20.** If the hospital where Mrs. S. planned to give birth did not have an intensive care nursery, the *best* course of action would have been to
   A. let her deliver at her chosen hospital but try to get the necessary emergency equipment that will be needed in the nursery before the baby is born
   B. let her deliver at her chosen hospital and hope the baby can survive with the care he receives from the available personnel and facilities
   C. let her deliver at her chosen hospital but have the special premature team from the nearest regional center present at the time of birth
   D. transfer her, before the baby is born, to a regional center that has an intensive care nursery

C 21. Of all the needs an individual is born with, those which are *least* likely to be met during the first few days of Baby S.'s life are his need for
  (1) food
  (2) adequate oxygenation
  (3) cuddling and love
  (4) warmth
  A. (1) and (2)
  B. (4) only
  C. (3) only
  D. All of these

A 22. Probably the most immediate concerns Mr. and Mrs. S. will have as a result of the premature birth of their son will be for
  (1) the life of their son
  (2) the health and normalcy of their son
  (3) the expense incurred
  (4) their ability to properly care for their son when he is discharged from the hospital
  A. (1) and (2)
  B. (2) and (4)
  C. (3) only
  D. (3) and (4)

D 23. If Mrs. S. is worried about her ability to care for Baby S. when she takes him home, probably the *best* way you can help her is to
  A. listen and let her express her fears to you
  B. tell her that when he goes home he will be very much like any other baby and won't need all the special equipment he needs now
  C. suggest that the visiting nurse check on him periodically after she gets him home
  D. arrange for her to come in and hold him and feed and care for him in the nursery several times before she takes him home

C 24. Nursing interventions to give support to the parents of a preterm infant include
  (1) arranging for them to see, touch or hold the infant
  (2) keeping them informed of his progress
  (3) explaining the equipment used in his care
  (4) involving them in his care as much as possible
  (5) being available to them after his discharge
  A. (1), (4), and (5)
  B. (2), (3), and (5)
  C. All of these
  D. All except (3)

II. Certain problems are associated with infants who are preterm, SGA, LGA, or post-term. In the space before the problem in Column I, place the letter of the type of infant who usually develops that problem, from Column II.

	I PROBLEM		II TYPE OF INFANT
A	**1.** Anemia	**A.**	Preterm
C	**2.** Congenital malformations	**B.**	Post-term
A D	**3.** Hyperbilirubinemia	**C.**	Small for gestational age (SGA)
D	**4.** Hypocalcemia	**D.**	Large for gestational age (LGA)
A C D	**5.** Hypoglycemia		
A	**6.** Hypothermia		
C	**7.** Intrauterine infections		
B	**8.** Meconium aspiration		
B	**9.** Neonatal asphyxia		
A D	**10.** Respiratory distress syndrome		
B	**11.** Unexplained intrauterine death		

III. **A.** In Column II below are the gestational ages in weeks for the infants listed in Column I. In Column III are the weights at birth for the same infants. In Column IV classify each infant as term, preterm, or post-term, according to its gestational age. In Column V classify each infant as average for gestational age (AGA), small for gestational age (SGA), or large for gestational age (LGA), according to its weight.

I Baby	II Weeks' gestation	III Birth weight		IV Classification by gestational age (term, preterm, post-term)	V Classification by weight (AGA, SGA, LGA)
		lb oz	grams		
1. Girl K.	28	2–15	1,332		
2. Girl E.	38	5–9	2,523		
3. Boy A.	39	6–10	3,005		
4. Boy W.	39	7–4	3,289		
5. Girl L.	36	3–15	1,786		
6. Boy F.	41	8–15½	4,068		
7. Girl P.	41	6–6	2,892		
8. Boy T.	39	7–9	3,430		
9. Boy M.	43	8–14	4,026		
10. Boy R.	38	4–13	2,183		

B. Which of the 10 infants above would be considered low birth weight?

I.
1. B
2. C
3. A
4. B
5. A
6. B
7. D
8. C
9. A
10. D
11. B
12. A
13. D
14. C
15. A
16. B
17. D
18. B
19. A
20. D
21. C
22. A
23. D
24. C

II.
1. A
2. C
3. A, D
4. D
5. A, C, D
6. A
7. C
8. B
9. B
10. A, D
11. B

III.

A.
1. preterm, AGA
2. term, AGA
3. term, AGA
4. term, AGA
5. preterm, SGA
6. term, LGA
7. term, AGA
8. term, AGA
9. post-term, AGA
10. term, SGA

B.
1. Girl K.
5. Girl L.
10. Boy R.